Fast Facts

Fast Facts: Diseases of the Pancreas and Biliary Tract

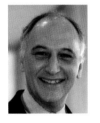

Jol MD FRCS
Professor of Surgery and ute of Cancer Studies,
University of Liverpool
Division of Surgery and Oncology
Royal Liverpool University Hospital
Liverpool, UK

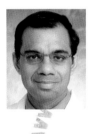

Manoop S Bhutani MD FACG FACP
Professor of Medicine
Co-Director, Center for Endoscopic Research, Training
and Innovation
Director, Center for Endoscopic Ultrasound
University of Texas Medical Branch
Galveston, Texas, USA

Declaration of Independence
This book is as balanced and as practical as we can make it.
Ideas for improvement are always welcome:
feedback@fastfacts.com

HEALTH PRESS

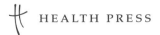

Fast Facts: Diseases of the Pancreas and Biliary Tract
First published March 2006

Text © 2006 John P Neoptolemos, Manoop S Bhutani
© 2006 in this edition Health Press Limited
Health Press Limited, Elizabeth House, Queen Street, Abingdon,
Oxford OX14 3LN, UK
Tel: +44 (0)1235 523233
Fax: +44 (0)1235 523238

Book orders can be placed by telephone or via the website.
For regional distributors or to order via the website, please go to:
www.fastfacts.com
For telephone orders, please call 01752 202301 (UK), +44 1752 202301 (Europe),
1 800 247 6553 (USA, toll free) or +1 419 281 1802 (Canada).

Fast Facts is a trademark of Health Press Limited.

The publisher and the authors have made every effort to ensure the accuracy of this
book, but cannot accept responsibility for any errors or omissions.

For all drugs, please consult the product labeling approved in your country for
prescribing information.

A CIP record for this title is available from the British Library.

ISBN 1-903734-74-6

Neoptolemos JP (John)
Fast Facts: Diseases of the Pancreas and Biliary Tract/
John P Neoptolemos, Manoop S Bhutani

Medical illustrations by Dee McLean, London, UK, and
Annamaria Dutto, Withernsea, UK.
Typesetting and page layout by Zed, Oxford, UK.
Printed by Fine Print (Services) Ltd, Oxford, UK.

Printed with vegetable inks on fully biodegradable and
recyclable paper manufactured from sustainable forests.

444   001
Low emissions
during production

Low
chlorine

Sustainable
forests

Glossary of abbreviations

AIDS: acquired immunodeficiency syndrome

ALT: alanine aminotransferase

APACHE: Acute Physiology And Chronic Health Evaluation

AST: aspartate aminotransferase

CA: cancer antigen

C_5A: complement $_5A$

CBD: common bile duct

CCK: cholecystokinin

CEA: carcinoembryonic antigen

CINC: cytokine-induced neutrophil chemoattractant

CFTR: cystic fibrosis transmembrane conductance regulator [gene]

CRP: C-reactive protein

CT: computed tomography

ENA: epithelial neutrophil-activating [protein]

ERCP: endoscopic retrograde cholangiopancreatography

EUS: endoscopic ultrasonography

5-FU: 5-fluorouracil

GGT: gamma-glutamyltransferase

GI: gastrointestinal

GRO: growth-related [protein]

HAART: highly active antiretroviral therapy

HIDA: hydroxyiminodiacetic acid

ICAM: intercellular adhesion molecule

IL: interleukin

MEN-1: multiple endocrine neoplasia type 1

MIBG: meta-iodobenzylguanide

MODS: multi-organ dysfunction syndrome

MRCP: magnetic resonance cholangiopancreatography

MRI: magnetic resonance imaging

NF-1: neurofibromatosis type 1

PAF: platelet-activating factor

PET: positron-emission tomography

PP: pancreatic polypeptide

PRSS1: protease serine 1 [gene]

PSC: primary sclerosing cholangitis

PSTI: pancreatic secretory trypsin inhibitor

SIRS: systemic inflammatory response syndrome

SPINK1: serine protease inhibitor, kazal type 1 [gene]

TNFα: tumor necrosis factor α

TSC: tuberous sclerosis

VHL: von Hippell–Lindau (syndrome)

VIP: vasoactive intestinal polypeptide

Introduction

The pancreas is important for the production of digestive enzymes (from the acinar cells), bicarbonate (from the duct cells) to neutralize gastric acid, and insulin (from the cells of the islets of Langerhans), essential for sugar control. It is the shape of a small flat fish, 6–8 inches long and salmon pink in color, and lies behind the stomach, stretching between the duodenum on the right to the center (hilum) of the spleen on the left (Figure 1). It is conventionally divided into the head, uncinate process, neck, body and tail.

The main pancreatic duct joins the bile duct to form the common channel or ampulla of Vater (also known as the major papilla or nipple). In 90% of people, the embryonic dorsal and ventral pancreatic ducts have fused to make this pancreatic duct, meeting in the head of the pancreas. In the other 10% the ducts drain separately into the duodenum (pancreas divisum), the dorsal duct (known as the accessory duct) draining through the minor papilla. Small sphincters around the

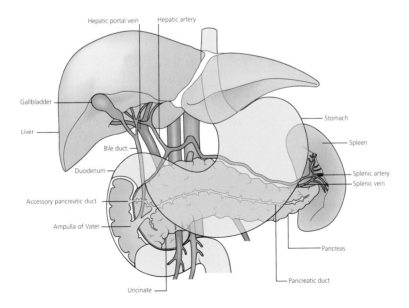

Figure 1 The anatomy of the pancreas and biliary tract.

ends of the main bile and pancreatic ducts control the flow of bile and pancreatic juice, respectively; the sphincter of Oddi controls the outflow from the ampulla of Vater.

Bile acids, essential for the absorption of fats and fat-soluble vitamins, are made in the liver and travel in canaliculi to reach the bile ducts. The intrahepatic bile ducts drain into the right and left hepatic ducts which fuse to form the common hepatic duct. The gallbladder is tucked under the right-hand side of the liver and is connected via the cystic duct to the common hepatic duct to become known as the common bile duct.

The various disorders of these systems will be encountered in any primary care practice. Gallstones are prevalent worldwide and a significant cause of morbidity and mortality. They may cause acute biliary colic, acute cholecystitis or chronic cholecystitis, acute pancreatitis or choledocholithiasis. Gallbladder carcinoma is the fifth most common gastrointestinal (GI) cancer in the USA and the most common GI cancer in Native Americans. Incidence and mortality are very high in certain Latin American countries, especially Chile. Bile duct cancer or cholangiocarcinoma may arise in the intra- or the extrahepatic biliary system, usually in those 50–70 years of age. Sclerosing cholangitis affecting the biliary system may occur in association with diseases such as ulcerative colitis and in secondary form due to conditions such as AIDS. The gallbladder and the biliary system may also be affected by dyskinetic conditions such as sphincter of Oddi dysfunction and gallbladder dyskinesia.

At least 45 000 North Americans will die every year from diseases of the pancreas, even excluding individuals with sugar diabetes. Each year 32 000 North Americans are newly affected with pancreatic cancer. Around 125 000 people in the USA will suffer an attack of acute pancreatitis each year and, separately, there are at least 100 000 long-term sufferers with chronic pancreatitis. All patients with pancreatic disease need to be seen and assessed by specialist doctors.

We have written this book with the intention of providing a clear and simple guide to the diagnosis and management of disorders of the pancreas and biliary tract. We hope that you will find that it helps you to help your patients.

Gallstones (cholelithiasis)

Etiology and pathogenesis. Gallstones are mainly composed of cholesterol, bilirubin and calcium salts. In Western populations, the majority of gallstones are the cholesterol type. These form when the cholesterol concentration in the bile exceeds the ability of bile to keep the cholesterol soluble by association with bile salts and phospholipids in the form of mixed micelles and vesicles. Non-cholesterol stones are black- or brown-pigmented stones made up of calcium salts of bilirubin. Black-pigmented stones are more common in patients with cirrhosis or chronic hemolytic states, whereas brown-pigmented stones occur more commonly as primary bile duct stones in association with infection.

Gallstones are a significant cause of morbidity and mortality worldwide. In the USA, gallstones occur in 5–8% of men and 13–26% of women. Native Americans have the highest prevalence in North America, with more than 70% of Pima Indian women having gallstones; African-Americans have the lowest prevalence. European studies have reported the prevalence of gallstones to be about 10% in men and about 20% in women, increased to 30% and 40% respectively in older patients.

Risk factors for gallstones. The prevalence of gallstones is greater in people over 40 years of age, and women are at higher risk than men. Other risk factors for gallstones are given in Table 1.1.

Symptoms and signs. Symptoms may arise from acute or chronic cholecystitis or choledocholithiasis (see Chapter 2, Bile duct stone disease). However, the majority of gallstones are asymptomatic and do not generally require treatment.

Some patients present without complications of gallstones but with mild symptoms of intermittent right upper quadrant pain (biliary colic). These patients are at increased risk for gallstone-related complications.

TABLE 1.1

Risk factors for gallstones

- Age > 40 years
- Female sex
- Estrogen replacement therapy
- Pregnancy
- Family history
- Obesity
- Diabetes mellitus
- Cirrhosis
- Crohn's disease
- Increased serum triglyceride levels
- Lack of exercise
- Drugs: octreotide, clofibrate, ceftriaxone
- Total parenteral nutrition
- Gastric bypass surgery

Diagnosis

Laboratory studies are generally normal in patients with uncomplicated or asymptomatic gallstones.

Plain abdominal radiography is usually unhelpful, as 85–90% of gallstones are radiolucent, but may reveal calcified gallstones in 10–15%; air in the biliary tree suggests a communication (fistula) between the gallbladder and bowel (usually the duodenum); air in the gallbladder wall and sometimes accompanied by an air–fluid level indicates emphysematous acute cholecystitis, often in association with diabetes mellitus; and rarely a calcified ('porcelain') gallbladder indicates a premalignant condition.

Abdominal ultrasound is the preferred test for diagnosis of gallstones. Gallstones characteristically have a highly echogenic focus with a typical acoustic shadow. The accuracy is 95–98%.

Endoscopic ultrasonography (EUS) is able to detect even small gallstones missed by regular abdominal ultrasound.

Magnetic resonance imaging (MRI) has an accuracy of 90–95% in detecting gallstones.

Computed tomography (CT) scan. Although CT scans, like MRI, are not the preferred test for the diagnosis of gallstones, gallstones may be detected in around 30% of patients when a CT scan is performed for other reasons, such as abdominal pain or jaundice.

Surgical treatment of gallstones. Surgical treatment of symptomatic gallstones and its major complications (acute cholecystitis, chronic cholecystitis, etc.) by cholecystectomy is the definitive treatment for gallstone disease, usually by the laparoscopic route.

Laparoscopic cholecystectomy. More than 700 000 laparoscopic cholecystectomies are performed annually in the USA. There are relatively few contraindications to laparoscopic cholecystectomy. They include severe coagulopathy, severe congestive heart failure and chronic obstructive pulmonary disease; patients with either of the latter two conditions may not tolerate the pneumoperitoneum needed for a laparoscopic cholecystectomy. Previous upper abdominal surgery may make the procedure difficult. Laparoscopic cholecystectomy can be performed in patients with well-compensated liver cirrhosis, although there is an increased risk of bleeding in some patients.

Conversion to an open operation is needed in about 5% of elective laparoscopic cholecystectomies, usually because anatomic landmarks cannot be seen clearly enough.

Most laparoscopic cholecystectomies are completed safely. Overall, the complication rate is 2.5% (comparable to that associated with open cholectystectomy). The main complications include bleeding, wound infection, bile leak, and injury to the bile duct. Less common complications include lacerations of the liver and bowel, pneumoperitoneum-related complications, intra-abdominal abscess due to inadvertent spillage of gallstones into the abdominal cavity, and retained common bile duct stones. The risk of biliary injury during laparoscopic cholecystectomy diminishes as the surgeon acquires experience and expertise.

Medical management of gallstones. Although cholecystectomy, usually by the laparoscopic route, remains the definitive treatment for gallstone disease, selected patients who are unfit for surgery for one reason or another may be candidates for medical therapy.

Bile acid treatment. Treatment options include ursodeoxycholic acid, which works by forming liquid cholesterol crystals, and chenodeoxycholic acid, which removes cholesterol as micelles.

This treatment is most successful for small stones in a normally functioning gallbladder and in the absence of acute cholecystitis. Prolonged treatment (up to 2 years) is usually required. Use of these agents may be limited by cost and side effects, notably diarrhea, and the recurrence rate is around 50% after 5 years.

Contact dissolution involves the use of solvents that dissolve gallstones on direct contact, but is now rarely used because of serious complications.

Extracorporeal shock-wave lithotripsy may be performed to destroy gallstones. It can be used on multiple stones, but is most effective for a single stone; the selection criteria to improve the results of the treatment are:

• solitary stone
• stone less than 2 cm in size
• normally functioning gallbladder
• non-obstructed cystic duct.

Bile acid therapy is combined with lithotripsy to promote clearance of stone fragments. Common complications of lithotripsy include biliary colic and pain. Less common complications include biliary obstruction, pancreatitis and injury to adjacent organs.

Acute cholecystitis

Etiology and pathogenesis. Acute cholecystitis caused by gallstones is in most cases due to obstruction of the cystic duct, which results in distension and inflammation of the gallbladder wall, which in turn may result in ischemia and necrosis. Inflammation and stasis may lead to secondary infection of bile. Severe cases may present with sepsis. Acalculous chlecystitis (see below) also occurs, notably as a complication of cardiac surgery.

Symptoms and signs. These include tenderness and guarding or pain in the right upper quadrant, nausea and vomiting, fever, fast pulse (tachycardia) and a positive Murphy's sign – transient cessation of breathing due to pain during inspiration while the right upper quadrant is palpated, but not the left upper quadrant. Complications include empyema, perforation of the gallbladder, liver abscess and emphysematous cholecystitis. An inflamed and distended gallbladder may obstruct the main bile duct by pressure from a gallstone causing obstructive jaundice (Mirizzi's syndrome).

Diagnosis

Laboratory studies. Leukocytosis and mild elevation in serum bilirubin and transaminases may be present.

Transabdominal ultrasound is the most useful test for acute cholecystitis as it establishes the presence of gallstones (Figure 1.1). A thickened gallbladder wall (> 4 mm) and pericholecystic fluid are highly suggestive of acute cholecystitis. Sonographic Murphy's sign – tenderness over the gallbladder from the ultrasound transducer during imaging – is also diagnostic.

Radionuclide scanning is a useful test if ultrasound is non-diagnostic or inconclusive but there is clinical suspicion of acute cholecystitis. A

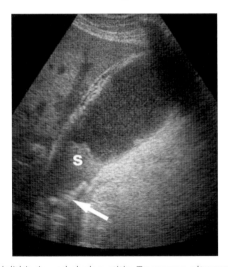

Figure 1.1 Cholelithiasis and cholecystitis. Transverse ultrasound imaging through the gallbladder demonstrating a distended gallbladder with sludge (S) and shadowing gallstones (arrow). Accompanying gallbladder wall thickening and minimal pericholecystic fluid, together with a positive sonographic Murphy's sign, are consistent with acute cholecystitis. Reproduced courtesy of Aytekin Oto MD, University of Texas Medical Branch.

^{99}Tc–HIDA (hydroxyiminodiacetic acid) scan uses a technetium-labeled analog of iminodiacetic acid. Non-visualization of the gallbladder with visualization of the tracer in the common bile duct and the small intestine is consistent with cystic duct obstruction. This test is about 95% accurate for the diagnosis of acute cholecystitis.

CT scanning is useful for identifying local complications of acute cholecystitis.

Treatment of acute cholecystitis involves:
- nothing by mouth
- intravenous fluids
- intravenous antibiotics
- analgesics.

Surgical treatment. The definitive treatment is cholecystectomy, which is usually attempted by the laparoscopic route, although conversion to open cholecystectomy may be needed in more than 30% of patients. Comparative studies of immediate (within 24–48 hours) versus delayed (after 6 weeks) laparoscopic cholecystectomy show similar rates for success, complications and conversion to open procedure. However, early laparoscopic cholecystectomy decreases hospital stay and medical costs. Subtotal cholecystectomy is sometimes needed if there is extensive inflammation and fibrosis around the gallbladder.

Chronic cholecystitis

Etiology and pathogenesis. Gallstones are the causative agent in the majority of patients with chronic cholecystitis. Recurrent or chronic obstruction of the cystic duct results in chronic inflammation of the gallbladder wall, which may lead to a non-functioning gallbladder. There is a small, long-term risk of developing gallbladder cancer.

Symptoms and signs include right upper quadrant and epigastric pain. Pain may be episodic and recurrent without the clinical features of acute cholecystitis, but constant right upper quadrant or epigastric pain is the more usual pattern in patients with chronic cholecystitis. Nausea and vomiting may occur when the pain is severe. Episodic pain may or may not be associated with meals, and right upper quadrant tenderness may or may not be present on physical examination. Common laboratory tests are usually normal.

Diagnosis is made when a patient with gallstones has the clinical signs and the symptoms with no other obvious cause.

Transabdominal ultrasound is the best test to demonstrate the presence of gallstones. Sludge is often seen in patients who have not eaten for at least a day and may be associated with other intra-abdominal illness, but is not of itself indicative of gallbladder disease. Thickening of the gallbladder wall may be seen in some patients.

Endoscopic ultrasound may be used in patients with chronic biliary-type pain but no gallstones on transabdominal ultrasound. EUS may demonstrate microlithiasis (gallstones that are 3 mm or less in size and usually do not cast an acoustic shadow).

Dynamic HIDA scan may be performed in selected patients with suspected gallbladder dysfunction when no gallstones or microlithiasis can be proven or if the symptoms are unusual.

A low gallbladder ejection fraction on gallbladder stimulation (fatty sandwich, 'Mars bar' [candy bar] or cholecystokinin [CCK] injection) and scan is consistent with the dysfunctional gallbladder that occurs in chronic cholecystitis. Reproduction of the patient's pain during the test may help establish a biliary cause of pain in atypical cases.

Treatment is by laparoscopic cholecystectomy. Conversion to open cholecystectomy is required in about 5% of patients.

Acalculous cholecystitis

This is an acute inflammatory condition that occurs in patients without gallstones. Stasis and ischemia are considered to be underlying pathophysiological factors. Acalculous cholecystitis may lead to perforation of the gallbladder.

Symptoms and signs. Acalculous cholecystitis is associated with a myriad of clinical conditions as predisposing factors, including:

- surgery
- sepsis
- shock
- total parenteral nutrition
- ventilator support
- trauma
- diabetes mellitus
- severe infections
- critical illness managed in the intensive care unit.

The usual scenario consists of abdominal pain, fever and leukocytosis in a patient with one of the predisposing conditions. Diagnosis requires a high index of suspicion. Right upper quadrant tenderness and Murphy's sign may be present, and a palpable mass may be detected in a minority of patients. Jaundice is not uncommon.

Abnormal laboratory tests may include leukocytosis, abnormal transaminases, hyperbilirubinemia and increased alkaline phosphatase levels.

Diagnosis

Plain abdominal radiography is useful to identify emphysematous cholecystitis, gas in the gallbladder and free air in the abdomen resulting from a perforated gallbladder.

Transabdominal ultrasound is the test of choice and can be done at the bedside in critically ill patients. Abdominal ultrasound may reveal thickening of the gallbladder wall, with pericholecystic fluid but no gallstones. Perforation of the gallbladder, abscess in the gallbladder fossa or air in the gallbladder wall may also be seen on ultrasound.

HIDA scanning may be used in selected cases if abdominal ultrasound is inconclusive. Non-visualization of the gallbladder is diagnostic of acute cholecystitis, but false-positive HIDA findings may occur in a variety of conditions.

CT scanning may show gallbladder inflammation, pericholecystic fluid or empyema of the gallbladder (Figure 1.2).

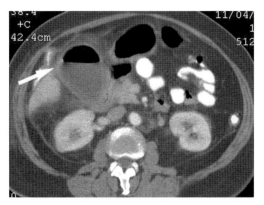

Figure 1.2 This axial contrast-enhanced computed tomography image shows a thick-walled gallbladder with an air–fluid level consistent with empyema of the gallbladder (arrow). Reproduced courtesy of Aytekin Oto MD, University of Texas Medical Branch.

Treatment. Patients require intravenous antibiotics. The treatment of choice is cholecystectomy; it may be attempted laparoscopically, but conversion to the open route may be needed. Percutaneous cholecystostomy may be considered as a temporary measure in patients who are too ill to undergo cholecystectomy. The disease has a high mortality, which is influenced significantly by the patient's underlying condition.

Gallbladder polyps

Epidemiology and pathogenesis. Gallbladder polyps are seen in about 5% of normal subjects undergoing gallbladder ultrasonography. Differential diagnosis of polypoid lesions of the gallbladder includes cholesterol polyps, adenomyomatoses, inflammatory polyps, adenomas and gallbladder carcinoma.

The clinical significance relates to the malignant potential of some of the polyps. Risk factors that increase the chance of malignancy in a gallbladder polyp include:

- size > 1 cm
- presence of gallstones
- age > 60 years
- increase in size on interval imaging.

Symptoms and signs. Most patients with gallbladder polyps are asymptomatic, discovery usually being incidental on imaging studies, although some patients may present with chronic and recurrent biliary-type pain.

Diagnosis

Transabdominal ultrasound. Gallbladder polyps are easily visualized on transabdominal ultrasound. The size and echo features of the polyp(s) assist in differential diagnosis and determination of malignant potential (> 1 cm in size is significantly associated with presence of malignancy).

Cholesterol polyps may be multiple, are usually pedunculated and are hyperechoic but with no acoustic shadow. Adenomas are usually solitary, sessile and more isoechoic.

CT scanning is not useful for detecting or for the differential diagnosis of small gallbladder polyps. It is more useful as a preoperative staging technique if malignancy is suspected in a polypoid lesion of the gallbladder.

EUS is a more precise modality for gallbladder imaging than abdominal ultrasound, but is more invasive. Data from a few studies show better differentiation of neoplastic and non-neoplastic polyps than with abdominal ultrasound.

Treatment. Cholecystectomy is indicated for polyps greater than 1 cm in size, for polyps with associated gallstones and for patients with biliary symptoms.

Solitary, sessile polyps that are 5–10 mm in size are more likely to be neoplastic than are small multiple, pedunculated, hyperechoic polyps. Cholecystectomy should be considered if a neoplastic polyp is suspected.

Observation with serial imaging is an option for small polyps that are considered at low risk for neoplastic features; generally speaking, small, apparently benign polyps are best ignored. Polyps that increase in size on serial imaging are an indication for cholecystectomy.

Gallbladder carcinoma

Epidemiology and pathogenesis. Gallbladder carcinoma is the fifth most common gastrointestinal (GI) cancer in the USA and is the most common GI cancer in Native Americans. Incidence and mortality are very high in certain Latin American countries, especially Chile.

The risk factors for gallbladder cancer are outlined in Table 1.2. The majority of gallbladder cancers are adenocarcinomas.

Symptoms and signs include abdominal pain, usually in the right upper quadrant, weight loss, anorexia, nausea and vomiting, fever, obstructive jaundice from invasion of the bile duct, and duodenal obstruction.

The clinical presentation may mimic acute cholecystitis, chronic cholecystitis or biliary obstruction due to other benign or malignant causes. On examination, patients may have jaundice, right upper quadrant tenderness and a palpable mass in the right upper quadrant.

Laboratory abnormalities will depend on the clinical presentation of, for example, acute or chronic cholecystitis, biliary obstruction, anorexia, weight loss or malaise, without clinical evidence of cholecystitis or biliary obstruction.

Diagnosis

Abdominal ultrasound is the usual initial method for imaging the gallbladder. Ultrasonographic findings of gallbladder cancer include a mass in the gallbladder, significant thickening or irregularity of the gallbladder wall and evidence of loss of interface with the liver or invasion of the liver.

TABLE 1.2

Risk factors for gallbladder cancer

- Gallstones
- Choledochal cysts
- Porcelain gallbladder
- Gallbladder polyps
- Anomalous pancreatic biliary junction
- Chronic *Salmonella*-type gallbladder infection

The sensitivity of abdominal ultrasound for detecting or suggesting the diagnosis of gallbladder cancer may be more than 70% but its accuracy for regional and distant staging is limited – 50% or less.

CT *scanning* is useful for staging to detect liver invasion, lymphadenopathy and distant metastases (Figure 1.3).

Magnetic resonance imaging with magnetic resonance cholangiopancreatography may be useful in mapping the extent of a tumor. Vascular encasement, particularly of the portal vein, lymphadenopathy and the biliary tree can be visualized.

ERCP or percutaneous transhepatic cholangiography are not needed routinely unless the patient presents with obstructive jaundice requiring biliary decompression, without an obvious diagnosis of gallbladder cancer.

EUS is useful in regional staging of gallbladder cancer associated with lymph-node metastases and vascular invasion. It may also be helpful in differentiating benign from malignant polyps of the gallbladder.

Treatment and prognosis. The staging of gallbladder cancer is shown in Table 1.3.

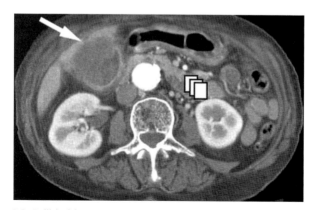

Figure 1.3 Gallbladder carcinoma. This axial contrast-enhanced computed tomography image reveals the enhancing soft tissue mass within the gallbladder (arrow); the rectangles indicate normal pancreas. Surgery confirmed the diagnosis of carcinoma of the gallbladder. Reproduced courtesy of Aytekin Oto MD, University of Texas Medical Branch.

TABLE 1.3

TNM staging of gallbladder cancer

T1	Tumor invades lamina propria (T1a) or muscle layer (T1b)
T2	Tumor invades perimuscular connective tissue
T3	Tumor perforates the serosa and/or directly invades the liver and/or one other adjacent organ or structure, such as stomach, duodenum, colon, or pancreas, omentum or extrahepatic bile ducts
T4	Tumor invades main portal vein or hepatic artery, or invades multiple extrahepatic organs or structures
Nx	Regional lymph nodes cannot be assessed
N0	No regional lymph-node metastases
N1	Regional lymph-node metastases
Mx	Distant metastases cannot be assessed
M0	No distant metastases
M1	Distant metastases

Stage grouping

IA	T1, N0, M0
IB	T2, N0, M0
IIA	T3, N0, M0
IIB	T1 or T2 or T3, N1, M0
III	T4, any N, M0
IV	any T, any N, M1

TNM, primary tumor, regional nodes, metastasis.

T1 lesions are usually found incidentally during cholecystectomy and are associated with a 5-year survival of more than 85%.

T1b patients have increased risk of lymph-node metastases. Many surgeons prefer reoperation with radical resection to maximize survival. T2 lesions should also be considered for radical resection.

Some surgeons recommend that a staging laparoscopy is performed before attempting surgical resection of known or suspected gallbladder cancer.

Radical resection with an extended cholecystectomy should be performed for stages II and III. Radical surgery for T3 or T4 disease has become more popular recently and may involve hepatic, pancreatic, duodenal and colonic resection. A hepatic lobectomy may be needed for anatomic reasons in some patients.

Treatment of unresectable disease with palliative chemotherapy and radiation therapy should be considered. Gemcitabine, cisplatin and 5-fluorouracil may be used for palliation, but only limited success has been achieved, and there are no firm recommendations. Radiation therapy using external-beam radiation has had limited effect in patients with unresectable tumors. Palliation for jaundice and bowel obstruction may involve surgical or endoscopic methods.

Prognosis and survival depend on the stage of the disease, and range from nearly 100% for T1a, 75% for T1b, 50–60% for T2 and 25–63% for stage IIA and IIB. Most patients who have unresectable tumors at the time of diagnosis have a 5-year survival of less than 15–20%.

Future trends
In the future we may hope for:
- Multimodal treatment approaches for gallbladder cancer
- Novel biological therapies
- Cancer vaccines and gene therapy
- Improved non-invasive and minimally invasive imaging techniques.

Key points – diseases of the gallbladder

- The prevalence of gallstones is greater in people over 40 years of age, and women are at higher risk than men.
- A ^{99}Tc–HIDA scan is 95% accurate for the diagnosis of acute cholecystitis.
- Acalculous cholecystitis may occur in critically ill patients; the diagnosis requires a high index of suspicion.
- Patients with gallbladder polyps of > 1 cm in size should be considered for cholecystectomy owing to the increased risk of malignancy.
- Gallbladder cancer is the most common GI cancer in native Americans in the USA and also has a very high incidence in certain Latin American countries, particularly Chile.

Key references

Chapman BA, Wilson IR, Frampton CM et al. Prevalence of gallbladder disease in diabetes mellitus. *Dig Dis Sci* 1996;41:2222–8.

Chijiiwa K, Nakano K, Ueda J, Noshiro H. Surgical treatment of patients with T2 gallbladder carcinoma invading the subserosal layer. *J Am Coll Surg* 2001;192: 600–7.

Dion YM, Morin J. The role of extracorporeal shock-wave lithotripsy in the treatment of symptomatic cholelithiasis. *Can J Surg* 1995;38:162–7.

Everhart JE, Yeh F, Lee ET et al. Prevalence of gallbladder disease in American Indian populations: Findings from the Strong Heart Study. *Hepatology* 2002;35:1507–12.

Fromm H, Malavolti M. Bile acid dissolution therapy of gallbladder stones. *Baillieres Clin Gastroenterol* 1992;6:689–95.

Greene FL, Page DL, Fleming ID et al, eds. *AJCC (American Joint Committee on Cancer) Cancer Staging Manual*, 6th edn. New York: Springer, 2002:139–149.

Manfredi S, Benhamiche AM, Isambert N, Prost P. Trends in incidence and management of gallbladder carcinoma: a population-based study in France. *Cancer* 2000;89:757–62.

Misra S, Chaturvedi A, Misra NC, Sharma ID. Carcinoma of the gallbladder. *Lancet Oncol* 2003; 4:167–76.

Nakamura S, Sakoguchi S, Suzuki S, Muro H. Aggressive surgery for carcinoma of the gallbladder. *Surgery* 1989;106:467–73.

Ohtani T, Shirai Y, Tsukada K, Muto T. Spread of gallbladder carcinoma: CT evaluation with pathologic correlation. *Abdom Imaging* 1996; 21:195–201.

Pandey M, Sood BP, Shukla RC, Aryya NC. Carcinoma of the gallbladder: role of sonography in diagnosis and staging. *J Clin Ultrasound* 2000;28:227–32.

Portincasa P, van de Meeberg P, van Erpecum KJ et al. An update on the pathogenesis and treatment of cholesterol gallstones. *Scand J Gastroenterol Suppl* 1997;223:60–9.

Rubin RA, Kowalski TE, Khandelwal M, Malet PF. Ursodiol for hepatobiliary disorders. *Ann Intern Med* 1994;121:207–18.

Shapiro MJ, Luchtefeld WB, Kurzweil S et al. Acute acalculous cholecystitis in the critically ill. *Am Surg* 1994;60:335–9.

Shiffman ML, Sugarman HJ, Kellum JM, Moore EW. Changes in gallbladder bile composition following gallstone formation and weight reduction. *Gastroenterology* 1992:103:214–21.

Strom BL, Soloway RD, Rios-Dalenz JL, Rodriguez-Martinez HA. Risk factors for gallbladder cancer. An international collaborative case-control study. *Cancer* 1995;76: 1747–56.

Sugiyama M, Atomi Y, Yamato T. Endoscopic ultrasonography for differential diagnosis of polypoid gall bladder lesions: Analysis in surgical and follow up series. *Gut* 2000; 46:250–4.

Terzi C, Sokmen S, Seckin S et al. Polypoid lesions of the gallbladder: Report of 100 cases with special reference to operative indications. *Surgery* 2000;127:622–7.

Torres WE, Steinberg HV, Davis RC et al. Extracorporeal shock wave lithotripsy of gallstones: Results and 6-month follow-up in 141 patients. *Radiology* 1991;178:509–12.

Yang HL, Sun YG, Wang Z. Polypoid lesions of the gallbladder: Diagosis and indications for surgery. *Br J Surg* 1992;79:227–9.

2 Bile duct stone disease (choledocholithiasis)

Epidemiology and pathogenesis

Stones within the common bile duct (CBD) are usually formed in the gallbladder and pass on to the CBD. They may be of the cholesterol or hard black-pigmented type (see Chapter 1, Diseases of the gallbladder). Primary stones form within the bile duct and are commonly of the soft brown-pigmented type; they are promoted by stasis.

Around 10% of younger patients with stones in the gallbladder have CBD stones at the time of cholecystectomy, rising with age to around 20%.

Clinical features

Symptoms include right upper quadrant pain, jaundice, clay-colored stools and dark urine. Cholangitis may be present, with fever, chills and right upper quadrant pain.

Signs include jaundice, fever and right upper quadrant tenderness. The presence of intermittent fever, jaundice and right upper quadrant pain (Charcot's triad) indicates infection of the bile ducts (acute cholangitis). Shock may also be present, with hypertension and tachycardia.

Diagnosis

Laboratory evaluation may reveal elevated serum levels of bilirubin, alkaline phosphatase, gamma-glutamyltransferase, aspartate aminotransferase and alanine aminotransferase, although these tests may occasionally be normal in patients with CBD stones. Leukocytosis is seen in patients with cholangitis.

Transabdominal ultrasound is non-invasive and is generally the first imaging modality used when a stone in the CBD is suspected. Its sensitivity for detection of a dilated bile duct is 55–90%, and higher in jaundiced patients. Its sensitivity for detection of stones in the CBD is lower, about 25%.

Endoscopic ultrasound (EUS) is a minimally invasive endoscopic imaging modality for CBD stones with an accuracy of around 98% and is now the preferred method of investigation. Intraductal ultrasound during endoscopic retrograde cholangiopancreatography (ERCP) has a similar accuracy and is marginally superior to ERCP alone. These diagnostic ERCP techniques are invasive and should generally not be used in preference to conventional EUS.

Magnetic resonance cholangiopancreatography (MRCP) is a non-invasive technique for imaging the extra- and intrahepatic biliary system (Figure 2.1). Contraindications include claustrophobia and implanted metal devices and fragments. MRCP is a useful and a reliable test for CBD stones but its accuracy is not quite as good as that of EUS. Most of the stones missed by MRCP are less than 6 mm in diameter.

Computed tomography cholangiography involves imaging the biliary ductal system after injection of contrast medium. The accuracy for CBD stones is around 85% less than that of either of EUS or MRCP.

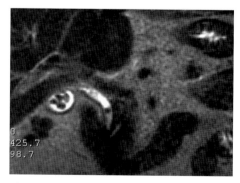

Figure 2.1 Thin-slice (5 mm) single-shot fast-spin echo coronal magnetic resonance cholangiopancreatography sequence showing a small filling defect in the mid-common bile duct. Multiple stones in the gallbladder and a normal-sized pancreatic duct near the ampulla can also be seen. Reproduced courtesy of Aytekin Oto MD, University of Texas Medical Branch.

ERCP is accurate in more than 90% of patients but should be performed only as a preliminary to therapeutic intervention. ERCP is more invasive than other imaging modalities, with risks that include acute pancreatitis (about 5%), bleeding and perforation.

Intraoperative cholangiography is performed at the time of cholecystectomy for the presence of CBD stones. It is performed routinely at some institutions, whereas others perform it when there is suspicion of retained CBD stones. In an analysis of more than 4000 patients undergoing laparoscopic cholecystectomy, 4% of patients were found to have stones in the CBD, but small stones do sometimes pass spontaneously from the CBD into the duodenum.

Choice of diagnostic test

Suspected choledocholithiasis in a patient with an intact gallbladder. When there is a high suspicion for the presence of a CBD stone on the basis of symptoms, signs, laboratory tests and abdominal ultrasound, one may proceed directly to ERCP, but in general EUS or MRCP should be performed as a prelude. If the preliminary examination proves negative then a cholecystectomy may be undertaken with the option of performing an intraoperative cholangiogram.

Suspected choledocholithiasis in postcholecystectomy patients. If there is high suspicion for CBD stones, one may proceed directly to ERCP, but again, in general, the diagnosis should first be confirmed by EUS or MRCP. Patients for whom the suspicion of CBD stones is low may be observed clinically for a while before initiating any investigation involving EUS or MRCP.

Treatment of choledocholithiasis

Any patient with obstructive jaundice, irrespective of the cause, is at risk of increased bleeding owing to malabsorption of vitamin K (bile-acid-dependent), which is required by the liver to make clotting factors II, VII, XI and X. Thus, clotting times need to be checked in all patients. Fresh frozen plasma may be required to correct clotting immediately. All patients will need vitamin supplementation by parenteral injection and/or absorbable modified vitamin K by mouth.

Cholangitis with choledocholithiasis. Cholangitis may be acute or chronic and is caused by at least partial obstruction to bile flow. Patients with acute cholangitis may have pain and tenderness in the right upper quadrant, jaundice and fever spikes (> 38°C) with chills – Charcot's triad. These patients usually respond to intravenous fluids and antibiotics, but subsequent clearance of CBD obstruction from stones is needed.

In severe or suppurative cholangitis, patients are severely ill, with septicemia, shock and mental confusion. Treatment with intravenous fluids and antibiotics may have to be supplemented by intensive care and vasopressors. Endoscopic biliary decompression by ERCP must be performed as an emergency and, if it is unsuccessful, radiological biliary intervention is required. Surgical intervention is associated with a high mortality and should be undertaken only when other methods have failed.

Endoscopic treatment. ERCP with sphincterotomy allows endoscopic extraction of stones from the CBD. If the ERCP clears all stones from the CBD, the patient can then undergo laparascopic cholecystectomy. Some patients may require more than one attempt by ERCP to clear all stones from the CBD. A plastic stent is sometimes placed in the bile duct during ERCP to achieve biliary drainage if not all stones can be removed and further attempts are planned. Large stones may require endoscopic lithotripsy during ERCP or extracorporeal lithotripsy in combination with ERCP.

Clearance of the CBD of all stones via ERCP is possible in more than 95% of patients. ERCP with sphincterotomy is also useful for patients who have recently undergone a cholecystectomy and present with retained CBD stones.

Complications of ERCP include pancreatitis, perforation, bleeding and cholangitis in about 5% of patients. The risk of cholangitis after ERCP is increased if ERCP is attempted but biliary drainage is not achieved. Thus, only physicians trained in therapeutic ERCP should attempt it. Alternative radiological and surgical methods for biliary decompression in acutely ill patients with biliary obstruction should be readily available.

Surgical management of choledocholithiasis. Cholecystectomy is recommended after ERCP with sphincterotomy and bile duct stone clearance, in order to prevent recurrence of biliary symptoms and biliary colic. Surgical exploration of the CBD may be needed for patients with CBD stones that could not be cleared by ERCP. Other indications for surgical CBD exploration include CBD stones discovered during intraoperative cholangiography.

Laparoscopic CBD exploration is performed through either the cystic duct or a choledochotomy (requiring postoperative T-tube drainage). This approach is successful in clearing CBD stones in more then 90% of cases.

Open CBD procedures are rarely performed nowadays but may occasionally be required when other non-surgical or laparoscopic methods are unsuccessful or impossible.

Key points – bile duct stone disease (choledocholithiasis)

- Around 10–20% of patients with stones in the gallbladder have common bile duct (CBD) stones at the time of cholecystectomy (the prevalence rises with age).
- Transabdominal ultrasound is only 25% accurate for detection of CBD stones.
- Endoscopic ultrasonography and magnetic resonance cholangiopancreatography are accurate, minimally invasive and non-invasive tests for detection of stones in the CBD and should generally precede endoscopic retrograde cholangiopancreatography (ERCP) unless the clinical signs and symptoms and abdominal ultrasound findings make a therapeutic ERCP inevitable.
- Clearance of the CBD of all stones via ERCP is possible in more than 95% of patients.
- Biliary decompression, preferably by endoscopic or radiologic means, is critical in severe suppurative cholangitis with choledocholithiasis.

Future trends

- More widespread application of non-invasive and minimally invasive imaging with MRCP and EUS.
- More clear-cut guidelines on use of various imaging modalities for detection of bile duct stones.

Key references

Eisen GM, Dominitz JA, Farigel DO et al. An annotated algorithm for the evaluation of choledocholithiasis. *Gastrointest Endosc* 2001;53: 864–6.

Ko CW, Lee SP. Epidemiology and natural history of common bile duct stones and prediction of disease. *Gastrointest Endosc* 2002;56(suppl 6):S165–9.

Napoleon B, Dumortier J, Keriven-Souquet O et al. Do normal findings at biliary endoscopic ultrasonography obviate the need for endoscopic retrograde cholangiography in patients with suspicion of common bile duct stone? A prospective follow-up study of 238 patients. *Endoscopy* 2003;35:411–15.

NIH Consensus conference. Gallstones and laparoscopic cholecystectomy. *JAMA* 1993; 269:1018–24.

NIH state-of-the-science statement on endoscopic retrograde cholangiopancreatography (ERCP) for diagnosis and therapy. *NIH Consens State Sci Statements* 2002; 19:1–26.

Pasanen PA, Partanen KP, Pikkarainen PH et al. A comparison of ultrasound, computed tomography and endoscopic retrograde cholangiopancreatography in the differential diagnosis of benign and malignant jaundice and cholestasis. *Eur J Surg* 1993;159:23–9.

Scheiman JM, Carlos RC, Barnett JL et al. Can endoscopic ultrasound or magnetic resonance cholangiopancreatography replace ERCP in patients with suspected biliary disease? A prospective trial and cost analysis. *Am J Gastroenterol* 2001;96:2900–4.

Yusuf TE, Bhutani MS. Role of endoscopic ultrasonography in diseases of the extrahepatic biliary system. *J Gastroenterol Hepatol* 2004;19:243–50.

Cholangiocarcinoma

Epidemiology and pathogenesis. Bile duct cancer or cholangio-carcinoma may arise in the intra- or the extrahepatic biliary system. It occurs predominantly in patients aged 50–70 years and is more common in men than women. The risk factors for cholangiocarcinoma are shown in Table 3.1. Adenocarcinoma is the most common histological type; molecular changes include the expression of mutant *p53* and *K-RAS*.

The bifurcation of the hepatic duct is the most common site for cholangiocarcinomas (Klatskin's tumor). Adenocarcinoma is the most common histological type.

Clinical features include obstructive jaundice, pruritus, right upper quadrant pain, weight loss, fever, acholic (pale) stools, dark urine and hepatomegaly. A right upper quadrant mass may be present.

Diagnosis. Laboratory findings include increased levels of bilirubin, alkaline phosphatase, aspartate aminotransferase, alanine aminotransferase and gamma-glutamyltransferase.

TABLE 3.1

Risk factors for cholangiocarcinoma

- Primary sclerosing cholangitis
- Choledochal cysts
- Liver flukes
- Oriental cholangiohepatitis
- Toxins (thorium dioxide contrast medium, rubber and other chemicals)
- Biliary papillomatosis

The serum tumor markers carcinoembryonic antigen (CEA) and cancer antigen (CA) 19.9 are usually elevated, but these may also indicate other types of tumor, and anyway may be mildly or moderately elevated in benign bilary obstruction.

Imaging. Transabdominal ultrasound is the first investigation indicating the level of biliary obstruction and sometimes the tumor mass itself.

Computed tomography (CT) will usually show the position and extent of the hilar cholangiocarcinoma along with a dilated intrahepatic biliary system with a non-dilated intrahepatic biliary tree and a non-dilated gallbladder. A CT scan of a distal bile duct cancer will show dilation of the intra- and extrahepatic biliary systems and the gallbladder. CT scans have limited ability to determine the resectability and extent of a tumor and often need to be supplemented by additional techniques.

Magnetic resonance cholangiopancreatography (MRCP) may provide supplementary definition of both the tumor and extent of biliary obstruction (Figures 3.1 and 3.2).

Endoscopic retrograde cholangiopancreatography (ERCP) or percutaneous transhepatic cholangiography is performed to obtain a diagnosis by brush cytology and permit temporary or permanent biliary decompression by means of a plastic or metal mesh stent, respectively.

Other imaging modalities include positron-emission tomography, endoscopic ultrasound and laparoscopic ultrasound, which may be useful adjuncts for establishing and defining the location and extent of a tumor.

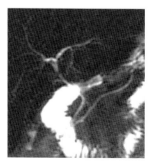

Figure 3.1 Thick-slab (2.5 cm) single-shot fast-spin echo coronal magnetic resonance cholangiopancreatography sequence demonstrating a normal common bile duct and pancreatic duct. Reproduced courtesy of Aytekin Oto MD, University of Texas Medical Branch.

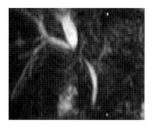

Figure 3.2 Three-dimensional magnetic resonance cholangiopancreatography (MRCP) image (reconstructed by maximum-intensity
projection algorithm from three-dimensional fast-spin echo
MRCP images) showing dilation of the right and left hepatic ducts
secondary to a malignant stricture in the proximal common bile duct.
The common bile duct distal to the tumor is normal. Reproduced courtesy
of Aytekin Oto MD, University of Texas Medical Branch.

Staging and classification. Perihilar cholangiocarcinoma is classified
according to the Bismuth classification, illustrated in Figure 3.3 and
summarized in Table 3.2.

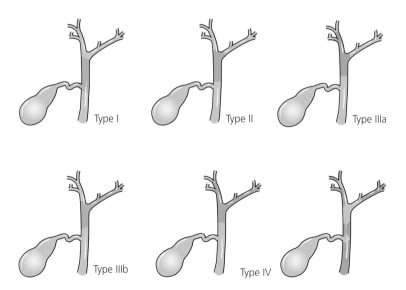

Figure 3.3 Bismuth classification of perihilar cholangiocarcinoma (see also
Table 3.2). (See De Groen et al. *N Engl J Med* 1999;341:1368–78.)

TABLE 3.2

The Bismuth classification and staging of perihilar cholangiocarcinoma

Type	Description of tumor (Figure 3.3)
I	Confined to the common hepatic duct
II	Involving the hepatic bifurcation but not the secondary intrahepatic ducts
IIIA	Involving the hepatic bifurcation and the right secondary intrahepatic ducts
IIIB	Involving the hepatic bifurcation and the left secondary intrahepatic ducts
IV	Involving the hepatic bifurcation and extending to both left and right secondary intrahepatic ducts

Stage	
IA	Tumor involving only the bile duct
IB	Tumor involving periductal tissues
IIA	Locally advanced tumor that is devoid of lymph-node metastases
IIB	Locally advanced tumor with adjacent lymph-node metastases
III	Unresectable, locally advanced tumor
IV	Tumor with distant metastases

Treatment. Surgical cure is possible in only a small proportion of patients. The type of operation depends on the location of the tumor, as follows.

- A distal cholangiocarcinoma is treated with a partial pancreatoduodenectomy (Whipple's procedure).
- A hilar lesion may be treated by local resection but usually requires a partial hepatic resection; in either case a hepatico-jejunostomy is required to restore continuity of the biliary-enteric tract.
- Intrahepatic lesions are treated with hepatic resection.

Preoperative stenting for alleviation of biliary obstruction may avoid deterioration of liver function but increases the risk of cholangitis and other complications following resection, especially in hilar lesions.

The 5-year survival after surgical resection varies from 10% to 40%.

Palliation of unresectable tumors. Biliary drainage may be achieved in unresectable disease by stents placed endoscopically or radiologically. Stents may be plastic (removable) or expandable metallic stents (non-removable). The method and choice of stent insertion depends on the location of the tumor, local expertise, and whether unresectability has been clearly determined at the time of stent insertion.

The value of chemotherapy or radiation in prolonging survival has not been adequately established.

Randomized studies using local photodynamic therapy have demonstrated prolonged biliary patency and survival.

Other bile duct tumors

Table 3.3 lists the various bile duct tumors.

Biliary papillomatosis presents as tumorous papillary growth of the bile duct epithelium and is usually diffuse and multiple. A large amount of mucus is produced by the abnormal biliary epithelium, causing biliary obstruction with resultant cholestatic jaundice and cholangitis.

TABLE 3.3

Tumors of the bile duct

- Cholangiocarcinoma
- Biliary papilloma
- Biliary cystadenoma
- Non-Hodgkin's lymphoma
- MALT lymphoma
- Carcinoid tumor

- Granular cell tumor
- Teratoma
- Adenoma
- Adenomyoma
- Metastases

MALT, mucosa-associated lymphoid tissue.

A possible association between Caroli's disease and biliary papillomatosis has been reported.

Biliary cystadenoma is a rare tumor. Malignant degeneration does occur, but very little is known of the risk for this. Because of the risk for malignancy and recurrence, surgical treatment encompassing resection or complete enucleation is recommended over marsupialization.

Lymphoma of the bile duct. Primary non-Hodgkin's lymphoma may arise from the bile duct. Jaundice may occur due to a variety of causes, including direct hepatic involvement, compression of the bile ducts by lymph nodes, and tumor-related hemolysis. This tumor can occur between the first and seventh decades of life. The most common lymphoma subtype pattern is large-cell lymphoma. Treatment is variable and includes some combination of chemotherapy, radiation and surgery.

Future trends

- Improved understanding of causes and etiology; for example, cholangiocarcinoma has been associated with hepatitis C and its stem-cell origin is being investigated
- Better patient selection for liver transplantation for hilar cholangiocarcinoma
- Molecular markers for improved preoperative diagnosis, prognostication and treatment selection
- Novel biological therapies
- Cancer vaccines and gene therapy
- Bioabsorbable stents for palliation
- Improved and new local treatments: photodynamic therapy, high-intensity focused ultrasonography, etc.
- Improved imaging for preoperative diagnosis (e.g. positron-emission tomography, endoscopic ultrasonography with fine-needle aspiration)
- Improved methods for pain control and palliation in a minimally invasive manner.

Key points – bile duct tumors

- Bifurcation of the hepatic duct is the most common site for cholangiocarcinoma.
- Primary sclerosing cholangitis is a risk factor for the development of cholangiocarcinoma.
- Benign biliary obstruction may increase CA 19.9 levels.
- Biliary papillomatosis is a mucus-producing tumor with diffuse multiple papillary lesions.
- Rare tumors of the bile duct include biliary cystadenoma and primary non-Hodgkin's lymphoma.

Key references

Bismuth H, Nakache R, Diamond T. Management strategies in resection for hilar cholangiocarcinoma. *Ann Surg* 1992;215:31–8.

Burke EC, Jarnagin WR, Hochwald SN et al. Hilar cholangiocarcinoma: patterns of spread, the importance of hepatic resection for curative operation, and a presurgical clinical staging system. *Ann Surg* 1998; 228:385–94.

Cameron JL, Pitt HA, Zinner MJ et al. Management of proximal cholangiocarcinoma by surgical resection and radiotherapy. *Am J Surg* 1990;159:91–7; dicussion 97–8.

Hoang TV, Bluemke DA. Biliary papillomatosis: CT and MR findings. *J Comput Assist Tomogr* 1998; 22:671–2.

Holtkamp W, Reis HE. Papillomatosis of the bile ducts: papilloma carcinoma sequence. *Am J Gastroenterol* 1994;89:2253–5.

Joo Y-E, Park C-H, Lee W-S et al. Primary non-Hodgkin's lymphoma of the common bile duct presenting as obstructive jaundice. *J Gastroenterol* 2004;39:692–6.

Klempnauer J, Ridder GJ, VonWasielewski R et al. Resectional surgery of hilar cholangiocarcinoma: A multivariate analysis of prognostic factors. *J Clin Oncol* 1997;15: 947–54.

Koffron A, Rao S, Ferrario M, Abecassis M. Intrahepatic biliary cystadenoma: Role of cyst fluid analysis and surgical management in the laparascopic era. *Surgery* 2004;136:926–36.

Kraybill WG, Lee H, Picus J et al. Multidisciplinary treatment of biliary tract cancers. *J Surg Oncol* 1994;55:239–45.

Lillemoe KD, Cameron JL. Surgery for hilar cholangiocarcinoma: The Johns Hopkins approach. *J Hepatobiliary Pancreat Surg* 2000;7:115–21.

Nagino M, Minura Y, Kamiya J et al. Segmental liver resections for hilar cholangiocarcinoma. *Hepatogastroenterology* 1998;45: 7–13.

Nakeeb A, Pitt HA, Sohn TA et al. Cholangiocarcinoma. A spectrum of intrahepatic, perihilar and distal tumors. *Ann Surg* 1996;224: 463–73; discussion 473–5.

Todoroki T, Kawamoto T, Koike N et al. Radical resection of hilar bile duct carcinoma and predictors of survival. *Br J Surg* 2000;87:306–13.

Tsao JI, Nimura Y, Kamiya J et al. Management of hilar cholangiocarcinoma: comparison of an American and a Japanese experience. *Ann Surg* 2000;232: 166–74.

Cysts of the biliary tree

Cysts involving the biliary tree may be isolated or multiple. Cyst dilation of the biliary tree may be intrahepatic or extrahepatic (choledochal intrahepatic cyst). The incidence in Western countries varies from 1 in 100 000 to 1 in 150 000. Biliary cysts are more common in East Asian countries. The prevalence is at least threefold higher in women than in men.

Pathogenesis and classification. Cysts of the biliary tree may be congenital or acquired, and there may be a familial occurrence. Congenital cysts may be diagnosed in the prenatal period.

More than 70% of patients with choledochal cysts have an abnormal pancreatobiliary junction, with a long common channel. Biliary cysts are associated with an increased risk for cholangiocarcinoma.

The classification of biliary cysts is shown in Table 4.1.

TABLE 4.1
Classification of biliary cysts

Type I	Cystic or fusiform dilation of the extrahepatic biliary tree (most common)
Type II	Supraduodenal diverticulum of the extrahepatic biliary duct
Type III	Intradudoenal diverticulum or cystic dilation of the intraduodenal portion (choledochocele)
Type IVA	Multiple cysts in the extrahepatic and intraphepatic ducts
Type IVB	Multiple extrahepatic cysts without intrahepatic involvement
Type V	Isolated or multiple cystic dilations of the intrahepatic biliary tree without extrahepatic involvement

Clinical manifestations. The classic triad of pain, jaundice and an abdominal mass is seen in only 10% of patients and is most common in infants, who may also present with raised bilirubin or failure to thrive.

Common manifestations in adults include chronic, intermittent abdominal pain, intermittent jaundice and acute cholangitis. Less common manifestations include pancreatitis, biliary lithiasis and intraperitoneal rupture.

Diagnosis. Transabdominal ultrasound or computed tomography (CT) scan may suggest the diagnosis. Cholangiography is generally considered the best method for the evaluation and definition of cysts, and for identifying associated stones or malignancy. The cholangiogram may be performed endoscopically, percutaneously or intraoperatively.

Magnetic resonance cholangiopancreatography (MRCP) allows non-invasive preoperative evaluation of the biliary tree. Endoscopic ultrasound (EUS) is useful for extrahepatic biliary cysts, to delineate the anatomy and to rule out stones or a mass within the dilated duct.

Treatment. Type I and II choledochal cysts are treated with cholecystectomy, resection of the extrahepatic biliary duct and hepaticojejunostomy. Type III cysts may be treated endoscopically. Type IV cysts should be resected. Hepatic lobectomy may be considered for intrahepatic cysts limited to one lobe. Stenosis of the hepaticojejunostomy with its sequelae is the most common long-term complication of surgery. Surgery decreases, but does not eliminate, cancer risk.

Caroli's disease

Caroli's disease is a congenital condition in which there are multiple, segmental dilations of the intrahepatic bile ducts.

Pathogenesis. Caroli's disease is commonly associated with congenital hepatic fibrosis. It may also be associated with renal cysts. Familial cases have been described, and the gene responsible has been mapped to chromosome 6.

Stagnation of bile leads to cholelithiasis, and patients have an increased risk for cholangiocarcinoma.

Clinical features include bacterial cholangitis, hepatic abscess and portal hypertension, leading to varices and ascites. Pruritus may be present and there may be intermittent abdominal pain.

Diagnosis

Laboratory studies reveal elevated serum levels of alkaline phosphatase and bilirubin. There may be leukocytosis in the presence of cholangitis, and coagulopathy.

Imaging. Transabdominal ultrasound, endoscopic retrograde cholangiopancreatography (ERCP) or MRCP may be useful in demonstrating the ductal dilations of the intrahepatic biliary system.

Liver biopsy may be needed in some cases to demonstrate the presence of congenital hepatic fibrosis.

Treatment. Antibiotics, often prolonged courses, are required for cholangitis and sepsis.

Intrahepatic stones may be difficult to remove by ERCP. Extracorporeal shock-wave lithotripsy or intraductal electrohydraulic lithotripsy may be needed in some patients to clear intrahepatic stones, and cholangioscopic removal of intrahepatic stones may be successful in some patients. Dissolution therapy using ursodeoxycholic acid for a long period (approximately 2 years) may be a useful adjunct.

Partial hepatectomy may be performed in patients with disease limited to one lobe. Patients who develop end-stage portal hypertension may require liver transplantation.

Oriental cholangiohepatitis

Oriental cholangiohepatitis has features of biliary obstruction secondary to intrahepatic biliary pigmented stones, with biliary dilation and strictures.

Epidemiology and pathogenesis. Oriental cholangiohepatitis occurs in Far Eastern countries and in immigrants from the Far East to the West.

Prevalence peaks in the third and fourth decades and is similar in men and women.

The pathogenesis is incompletely understood. Formation of multiple pigmented stones in the intrahepatic bile ducts proximal to biliary strictures results in recurrent cholangitis. Strictures may also affect the extrahepatic biliary system. The left hepatic system is more commonly involved, but the reasons for this are unclear.

Biliary parasites have been implicated in the pathogenesis of Oriental cholangiohepatitis. Liver flukes (*Clonorchis sinensis, Opisthorchis felineus, O. viverrini, Fasciola hepatica, F. giganta*) and roundworms (*Ascaris lumbricoides*) are the parasites most commonly implicated in this disease. Bacterial infection and stasis further contribute to stone formation, structuring and infection.

Clinical features. Recurrent cholangitis occurs in 44% of patients, abdominal pain in 32% and pancreatitis (due to passage of a common bile duct stone) in 17%. Liver abscess, cirrhosis and rupture of biliary ducts, with fistula formation, may also occur.

Diagnosis

Transabdominal ultrasound may reveal bile duct dilation and stones. This is a useful initial test when the disease is clinically suspected.

CT may show dilated ducts, abscesses, stones or bilomas and may also be useful in mapping out the extent of the disease.

Cholangiography. An MRCP scan can provide detailed visualization of the biliary system non-invasively but no therapy is possible, whereas ERCP, although more invasive, allows therapeutic intervention. In difficult cases, percutaneous transhepatic cholangiography may be required to define the ductal system and intervene therapeutically.

Treatment. Treatment of acute cholangitis requires antibiotics and biliary drainage. Biliary drainage is more difficult in this disease than with other causes of biliary obstruction and may be achieved using endoscopic, radiological or surgical methods, depending on local expertise.

Cholangioscopy may be performed during ERCP or percutaneously and may allow dilation of strictures and lithotripsy. Stones recur in 30% of patients.

Surgery may involve cholecystectomy with common bile duct exploration and T-tube drainage; in a minority of patients (usually those with left hepatic disease), partial hepatic resection may be feasible.

Hepatic failure may occur due to cirrhosis. The risk of cholangiocarcinoma is 3–5%.

AIDS cholangiopathy

Epidemiology and pathogenesis. This disease causes biliary obstruction from strictures caused by opportunistic infections in patients with acquired immunodeficiency syndrome (AIDS). The organism most commonly implicated in AIDS cholangiopathy is *Cryptosporidium parvum*; microsporidium and cytomegalovirus have also been implicated.

Clinical features. Before the advent of highly active antiretroviral therapy (HAART), the prevalence of cholangiopathy in AIDS patients was about 25%. It usually occurs when the CD4 count is < 100/mm^3.

The most common manifestations are right upper quadrant pain and diarrhea; jaundice and fever also occur. Liver function tests reveal the cholestatic picture but may be normal in some patients.

Diagnosis

Transabdominal ultrasound is the initial screening procedure; if abnormal, further testing may be done to confirm the diagnosis.

ERCP allows the diagnosis to be confirmed and any indicated therapy performed. The most common findings on ERCP are sclerosing cholangitis and papillary stenosis (approximately 60%). Less commonly, either of these conditions may be found in isolation.

MRCP has not been widely evaluated in patients with AIDS cholangiopathy but maybe useful as a diagnostic test.

Treatment. Medical treatment for infection with a causative agent (if identified) does not usually affect progression of this disease.

In addition, AIDS cholangiopathy usually occurs in patients with advanced AIDS, and as such their survival is not likely to be determined by this condition.

Sphincterotomy may be performed in patients with papillary stenosis along with abdominal pain or jaundice and provides relief of pain in 23–70% of patients but does not change strictures in the biliary tree. It is not helpful in the absence of papillary stenosis.

Ursodeoxycholic acid may help a small percentage of patients.

Primary sclerosing cholangitis

In primary sclerosing cholangitis (PSC), fibrotic strictures occur in the intra- and extrahepatic biliary system, with no obvious cause.

Epidemiology and pathogenesis. Genetic and immunologic factors are important in the pathogenesis of PSC, and it is more common in B8/DR3 haplotypes. Ulcerative colitis is strongly associated with PSC – up to 70% of patients with PSC may have ulcerative colitis. Patients with PSC have an increased risk for cholangiocarcinoma, estimated at 1% per year. Biliary obstruction may cause secondary biliary cirrhosis and hepatic failure.

Clinical features. The natural history of PSC is variable. The mean age of presentation is between 40 and 50 years and the disease is more common in men than women.

Clinical features include pruritus, jaundice, fatigue and abnormal liver function tests. Patients may present with signs and symptoms of end-stage liver disease and portal hypertension.

Diagnosis

MRCP should be used as a non-invasive method to image the biliary tree.

ERCP. The diagnosis of PSC by ERCP also allows brushing and biopsy when cholangiocarcinoma is suspected.

Liver biopsy may be required in selected patients to assess the degree of liver fibrosis or to document the presence of cirrhosis in order to select appropriate therapy.

Treatment and prognosis. Median survival from the time of diagnosis is about 12 years. Ursodeoxycholic acid may decrease serum transaminases and bilirubin levels, but may not delay disease progression.

Surgical resection may be an option in patients with significant hepatic fibrosis without cirrhosis; it may involve resection of the extrahepatic biliary tree and hepaticojejunostomy. In patients without cirrhosis, 5-year survival is longer with surgical treatment (approximately 80%) than with non-surgical endoscopic treatment with sphincterotomy and balloon dilation of strictures (approximately 40%).

Liver transplantation is needed for patients with PSC and end-stage liver disease and has a 5-year survival rate of more than 80%.

Future trends

- More non-invasive cholangiographic imaging with MRCP rather than with ERCP
- Molecular markers to improve diagnosis of cholangiocarcinoma in PSC
- More trials with newer drugs such as tacrolimus for treatment.

Key points – unusual disorders of the biliary tree

- More than 70% of patients with choledochal cysts have an abnormal pancreatobiliary junction.
- Caroli's disease is a congential condition resulting in multiple, segmental dilations of intrahepatic ducts.
- Liver flukes and roundworms may cause Oriental cholangiohepatitis.
- AIDS cholangiopathy may result in right upper quadrant abdominal pain, biliary strictures and papillary stenosis.
- Up to 70% of patients with primary sclerosing cholangitis (PSC) may have ulcerative colitis.
- Liver transplantation is the treatment of choice for PSC with end-stage liver disease.

Key references

Ahrendt SA, Pitt HA, Kalloo AN et al. Primary sclerosing cholangitis: Resect, dilate or transplant? *Ann Surg* 1998;227:412–23.

Alonso-Lej F, Rever W, Pessagno DJ. Congenital choledochal cyst, with a report of 2 and an analysis of 94 cases. *Int Abstr Surg* 1959;108:1–30.

Cello JP. Acquired immunodeficiency syndrome cholangiopathy: Spectrum of disease. *Am J Med* 1989;86: 539–46.

Cello JP, Chan MF. Long-term follow-up of endoscopic retrograde cholangiopancreatography sphincterotomy for patients with acquired immune deficiency syndrome papillary stenosis. *Am J Med* 1995;99:600–3.

Chijiiwa K, Koga A. Surgical management and long-term follow-up of patients with choledochal cysts. *Am J Surg* 1993;165:238–42.

Lipsett PA, Pitt HA, Colombani PM et al. Choledochal cyst disease: A changing pattern of presentation. *Ann Surg* 1994;220:644–52.

Sherlock S. Overview of chronic cholestatic conditions in adults: terminology and definitions. *Clin Liver Dis* 1998;2:217–33.

Summerfield JA, Nagafuchi Y, Sherlock S et al. Hepatobiliary fibropolycystic diseases. A clinical and histological review of 51 patients. *J Hepatol* 1986;2:141–56.

Taylor AC, Palmer KR. Caroli's disease. *Eur J Gastroenterol Hepatol* 1998;10:105–8.

Todani T, Watanabe Y, Narusue M et al. Congenital bile duct cysts: Classification, operative procedures, and review of thirty-seven cases including cancer arising from choledochal cyst. *Am J Surg* 1977;134:263–9.

Dysfunctional disorders of the sphincter of Oddi complex and gallbladder

Sphincter of Oddi dysfunction

Pathogenesis. The sphincter of Oddi is a complex of circular and longitudinal muscle fibers that surrounds the biliary and pancreatic sphincters where they open into the duodenum. Disorders of the sphincter of Oddi may present as sphincter stenosis or dyskinesia. Sphincter of Oddi stenosis is an actual anatomic narrowing of the sphincter, caused by inflammation, pancreatitis, gallstone passage or other unusual causes. Sphincter dyskinesia on the other hand is a spastic functional disorder of the sphincter.

Clinical manifestations. Dysfunction mostly occurs after cholecystectomy but may occur in a patient with an intact gallbladder. It causes biliary-type pain and may present as recurrent pancreatitis.

Diagnosis and classification. The classification of the disorders of the biliary and pancreatic sphincter is listed in Table 5.1.

Sphincter of Oddi manometry is the diagnostic gold standard. The biliary and pancreatic duct pressures are measured; an elevated basal pressure above 40 mmHg is diagnostic. A decrease in basal pressure after administration of a smooth-muscle relaxant may help to differentiate between stenosis and spasm. The limitations of this test include its invasiveness, lack of availability and an increased risk of pancreatitis.

Cross-sectional imaging. Dilation of the common bile duct is seen on abdominal ultrasound. Endoscopic retrograde cholangio-pancreatography (ERCP) reveals dilation of the bile or pancreatic duct, and drainage of contrast medium from the biliary or pancreatic ductal systems is delayed.

Provocation tests. An increase in the size of the bile duct (by more than 2 mm) after injection of cholecystokinin or an increase in the size of the pancreatic duct (by more than 1.5 mm) after injection of

TABLE 5.1

Classification of biliary and pancreatic sphincter dysfunction

Features of biliary sphincter dysfunction

A   AST and ALT abnormal on at least two occasions and associated with abdominal pain

B   Dilated common bile duct on ultrasonography or ERCP

C   Delayed biliary drainage of contrast

Features of pancreatic sphincter dysfunction

A   Abdominal pain with increased pancreatic enzymes (> 1.5 times normal)

B   Dilated pancreatic duct on imaging

C   Delayed pancreatic duct drainage of contrast after ERCP

Classification

- Type I dysfunction is associated with all three features (A, B and C)
- Type II dysfunction is associated with one or two features
- Type III dysfunction has none of the features

ALT, alanine aminotransferase; AST, aspartate aminotransferase; ERCP, endoscopic retrograde cholangiopancreatography.

secretin supports the diagnosis of biliary or pancreatic sphincter dysfunction, respectively.

Hepatobiliary scintigraphy with technetium-99m may help establish the existence of delayed biliary drainage and may support a diagnosis of biliary sphincter dysfunction.

Treatment

Pharmacological treatment. A trial of smooth-muscle relaxants may be useful, but results vary, and benefit may not be sustained in the long term or may be limited by side effects. Calcium-channel blockers (nifedipine) and nitrates have also been tried. Oral nifedipine was found to relieve pain in patients who had previously undergone cholecystectomy and who had elevated basal pressure and sphincter of Oddi phasic contractions of predominantly antegrade nature.

Endoscopic treatment takes the form of biliary or pancreatic sphincterotomy during ERCP. Pancreatic sphincterotomy may be undertaken if recurrent pancreatitis is considered to be related to pancreatic sphincter hypertension. Underlying chronic pancreatitis may adversely affect the outcome of pancreatic sphincterotomy via surgical or endoscopic methods.

Patients with type I biliary sphincter dysfunction respond well to sphincterotomy, which can be performed without manometry of the biliary sphincter.

Sphincter of Oddi manometry should be considered to confirm a diagnosis of type II biliary dysfunction.

Type III biliary dysfunction is the hardest to treat, and there is no clear consensus on or understanding of invasive diagnostic procedures, treatment with sphincterotomy or the existence of other contributing or alternative causes of pain.

Surgery may enable a more complete biliary or pancreatic sphincterotomy, with decreased chances of recurrent stenosis, but is more invasive than endoscopic treatment.

Gallbladder dyskinesia

Pathogenesis. Gallbladder dyskinesia is a disorder caused by abnormal motility or contraction of the gallbladder in the absence of gallstones. Surgical resection of a dysfunctional, dyskinetic gallbladder reveals acalculous chronic cholecystitis in most patients.

Clinical features include intermittent right upper quadrant pain, often postprandially. Nausea and vomiting also occur, possibly related to intake of fatty food.

Diagnosis. Liver function tests and white cell count are normal. Abdominal ultrasonography shows a normal-sized common bile duct and no stones in the gallbladder. Other investigations (e.g. endoscopy and/or computed tomography scan) may be needed to rule out other causes of right upper quadrant pain.

Scintigraphy. A ^{99}Tc–HIDA scan (which uses a technetium-labeled analog of iminodiacetic acid) with gallbladder stimulation by a sandwich, a 'Mars bar' (candy bar) or intravenous administration of cholecystokinin (CCK) can be used to calculate the gallbladder ejection fraction; an ejection fraction below 35% is considered abnormal. In some patients the pain of gallbladder dyskinesia is reproduced when CCK is administered.

Treatment is by cholecystectomy, usually laparoscopic, which may result in improvement or resolution of pain in more than 80% of patients.

Future trends
- Improved understanding of pathophysiology and mechanisms causing pain in sphincter of Oddi dysfunction
- Improved understanding of other diseases and mechanisms causing pain that is similar or overlapping with pain from sphincter of Oddi dysfunction.

Key points – dysfunctional disorders of the sphincter of Oddi complex and gallbladder

- Sphincter of Oddi dysfunction may occur due to anatomic stenosis or as a spastic functional disorder.
- Sphincter of Oddi dysfunction is most common after cholecystectomy.
- Sphincter of Oddi manometry is the diagnostic 'gold standard' for the dysfunction.
- Biliary or pancreatic duct pressure of > 40 mmHg are diagnostic of biliary or pancreatic sphincter dysfunction, respectively.
- A low gallbladder ejection fraction of < 35% on ^{99}Tc–HIDA scan with cholecystokinin (CCK) administration may be diagnostic of gallbladder dyskinesia.
- In some patients the pain of gallbladder dyskinesia is reproduced when CCK is administered.

Key references

Botoman, VA, Kozarek RA, Novell LA et al. Long-term outcome after endoscopic sphincterotomy in patients with biliary colic and suspected sphincter of Oddi dysfunction. *Gastrointest Endosc* 1994;40:165–70.

Choudhry U, Ruffolo T, Jamidar P et al. Sphincter of Oddi dysfunction in patients with intact gallbladder: Therapeutic response to endoscopic sphincterotomy. *Gastrointest Endosc* 1993;39:492–5.

Chuttani R, Carr-Locke DL. Pathophysiology of the sphincter of Oddi. *Surg Clin North Am* 1993;73:1311–22.

Geenen JE, Hogan WJ, Dodds WJ et al. The efficacy of endoscopic sphincterotomy after cholecystectomy in patients with sphincter-of-Oddi dysfunction. *N Engl J Med* 1989;320:82–7.

Hogan WJ, Geenen JE. Biliary dyskinesia. *Endoscopy* 1988;20(suppl 1):179–83.

Khuroo MS, Zargar SA, Yattoo GN. Efficacy of nifedipine therapy in patients with sphincter of Oddi dysfunction: a prospective double-bind randomized, placebo-controlled cross over trial. *Br J Clin Pharmacol* 1992;33:477–85.

Neoptolemos JP, Bailey JS, Carr-Locke DL. Sphincter of Oddi dysfunction: results of treatment by endoscopic sphincterotomy. *Br J Surg* 1988;75:454–9.

Sherman S, Troiano FP, Hawes RH et al. Frequency of abnormal sphincter of Oddi manometry compared with the clinical suspicion of Oddi dysfunction. *Am J Gastroenterol* 1991;86:586–90.

Toouli, J. Sphincter of Oddi. *Gastroenterologist* 1996;4:44–53.

Epidemiology and natural history

Inherited abnormal genes play a strong part in the clinical manifestation of three distinct types of pancreatitis:

- hereditary pancreatitis
- idiopathic chronic pancreatitis
- alcohol-related chronic pancreatitis.

The genes responsible and their association with the different types of pancreatitis are outlined in Table 6.1.

Hereditary pancreatitis is transmitted in a Mendelian autosomal-dominant manner and often afflicts affected individuals with recurrent acute abdominal pain (pancreatitis) from a very young age. To make the diagnosis of hereditary pancreatitis there should be at least two first-degree relatives in two or more generations with proven chronic pancreatitis. The disease is apparent only in about 80% of individuals with a known causative gene – hence the term 80% penetrance. (The gene is silent in the other 20%.)

The nature of the abdominal pain is commonly misdiagnosed in children and young adults and this fact, coupled with the reduced penetrance, often leads to clinical confusion and a failure to identify the existence of close relatives with pancreatitis. The prevalence of hereditary pancreatitis, at least in Northern Europe, has been greatly underestimated; in fact it affects at least one family in every million in the general population.

By the age of 70 years, 60% of patients with hereditary pancreatitis will develop exocrine insufficiency, including all of the expected symptoms of steatorrhea and weight loss (Figure 6.1). By this age 70% will also develop diabetes mellitus, almost all of whom will require insulin (Figure 6.2). Exocrine and endocrine failure develop in a much higher proportion of patients with hereditary pancreatitis than those with either idiopathic or alcoholic pancreatitis, but the time to failure is longer (Table 6.2). By the age of 70 years, about 35% of patients are at

TABLE 6.1

Abnormal genes associated with inherited forms of chronic pancreatitis

Protease serine 1 (PRSS1) gene
- Also known as the *cationic trypsinogen* gene
- Main cause of hereditary pancreatitis
- Autosomal-dominant inheritance
- Mutations mainly at codons 122, 29 and 16
- More than 20 mutations have been described
- Mutations of *PRSS1* are found in up to 80% of families with hereditary pancreatitis but are very rare in the general population
- In affected families, the penetrance of the disease is about 80% (the disease is silent in the other 20%)

Cystic fibrosis transmembrane conductance regulator (CFTR) gene
- Autosomal-recessive inheritance
- Mutations or polymorphisms found in:
  - up to 5% in the general population
  - up to 20% of patients with alcohol-related chronic pancreatitis
  - over 50% of patients with idiopathic pancreatitis
- Compound heterozygotes are common (different mutations in each of the *CFTR* genes)
- One of more than 1000 different mutations or polymorphisms may be involved

Serine protease inhibitor, kazal type 1 (SPINK1) gene
- Also known as the *pancreatic secretory trypsin inhibitor (PSTI)* gene
- Autosomal-recessive inheritance
- Commonest mutation is N34S, found in:
  - 0.5–4% in the general population
  - about 10% of patients with alcohol-related chronic pancreatitis
  - up to 30% of patients with idiopathic pancreatitis
- The N34S mutation may be found clustered in families with a high incidence of pancreatitis, but the disease does not necessarily relate to the presence of the mutation

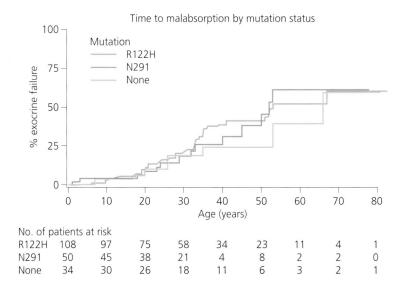

Figure 6.1 Cumulative incidence of pancreatic exocrine failure in hereditary pancreatitis according to *PRSS1* mutation status: R122H or N29I mutations or no mutation. Adapted from Howes et al. 2004.

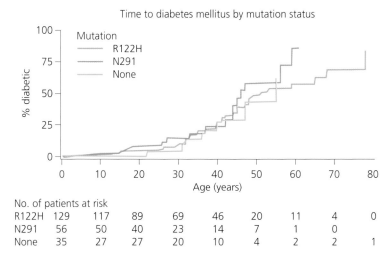

Figure 6.2 Cumulative incidence of pancreatic endocrine failure in hereditary pancreatitis according to *PRSS1* mutation status: R122H or N29I mutations or no mutation. Adapted from Howes et al. 2004.

TABLE 6.2

Characteristics of pancreatic exocrine and endocrine failure in hereditary, idiopathic and alcoholic pancreatitis

Type of pancreatitis	Cumulative exocrine failure	Time to exocrine failure	Cumulative diabetes mellitus	Time to diabetes mellitus
Hereditary	60%	53 years	69%	53 years
Early-onset idiopathic	44%	26 years	32%	28 years
Late-onset idiopathic	46%	17 years	41%	12 years
Alcoholic	48%	23 years	38%	20 years

risk of pancreatic cancer (Figure 6.3). This incidence is much higher than with other forms of chronic pancreatitis (estimated at around 5%) and compares with an incidence of 1% in the general population.

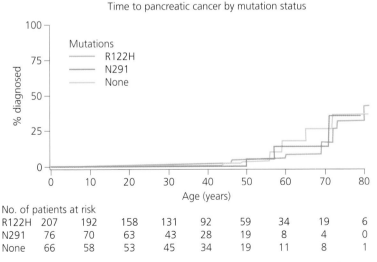

Figure 6.3 Cumulative incidence of pancreatic cancer in patients with hereditary pancreatitis according to *PRSS1* mutation status: R122H or N29I mutations or no mutation. Adapted from Howes et al. 2004.

Idiopathic pancreatitis has no apparent cause other than a genetic predisposition, which occurs in about 25% of patients with chronic pancreatitis. There are two types of idiopathic pancreatitis: the more common is early onset (child or young adult) whereas the other occurs in much older patients.

Alcoholic pancreatitis. About 70% of cases of chronic pancreatitis are associated with chronic excess alcohol consumption, but fewer than 10% of known alcoholics develop chronic pancreatitis. Whereas cumulative alcohol consumption is directly related to the development of liver cirrhosis, this is not the case in chronic alcoholic pancreatitis, which appears in general to be associated with a lower threshold of total alcohol consumed. About 10% of patients develop both liver cirrhosis and chronic pancreatitis. Inherited genetic factors are clearly involved but are incompletely understood.

Pathogenesis

The histological and radiological features of the three types of chronic pancreatitis are indistinguishable. Under physiological circumstances, pancreatic enzymes are released in a non-activated form (principally as proenzymes) from secretory granules in pancreatic acini into pancreatic ductules. Secretion is stimulated either by cholecystokinin (also known as pancreozymin) released from the duodenum upon entry of food, or by acetylcholine following neural stimulation. Normally, trypsinogen is activated to trypsin in the duodenal lumen by the action of enterokinase. Once activated, trypsin in turn activates all the other proenzymes in the pancreatic juice in the duodenal lumen. Trypsin also activates itself, resulting in exponential amplification of trypsin activity.

The mechanisms by which mutation in the *trypsinogen* and *SPINK1* (*serine protease inhibitor, kazal type 1*) genes result in inappropriate trypsin activity entirely within the pancreatic parenchyma are shown in Figure 6.4. Mutations in the *trypsinogen* gene result in spontaneous excess self-activation of trypsinogen or resistance to deactivating enzymes, or both. The first line of defense comprises collectively the deactivating enzymes – enzyme Y and meso-trypsin

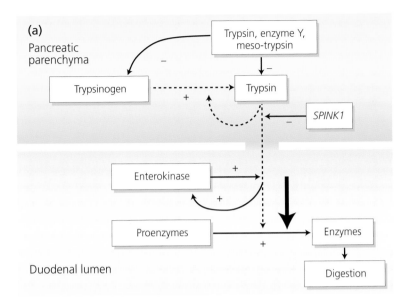

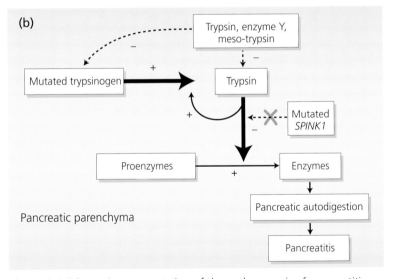

Figure 6.4 Schematic representation of the pathogenesis of pancreatitis secondary to mutations of either the *PRSS1* or *SPINK1* genes (Table 6.1). (a) The normal activation mechanism of trypsinogen to trypsin and the containment of inappropriately activated trypsin. (b) Gene mutations that affect either trypsinogen or SPINK1 result in inappropriate trypsinogen activation within the pancreatic parenchyma and thus pancreatitis.

(as well as trypsin); the second line of defense is SPINK1 protein. Once the first line of defense is breached, inactivation of trypsin is not possible if *SPINK1* is mutated.

The cystic fibrosis transmembrane conductance regulator (CFTR) protein moves chloride ions out of the pancreatic ductal cells into the pancreatic duct lumen in response to secretin hormone stimulation. A large movement of sodium and bicarbonate ions together with a large volume of water molecules accompanies the movement of chloride. This helps to wash the pancreatic enzymes into the duodenal lumen, and the bicarbonate counteracts the hydrogen ions in the gastric juice entering the duodenum. Thus, the pH of duodenal chyme is raised, which helps to optimize the activity of the digestive enzymes.

The CFTR protein is not produced in pancreatic acini, so it is not entirely clear how mutations of the *CFTR* gene also result in pancreatitis that is otherwise pathologically indistinguishable from any other type of pancreatitis.

Clinical presentation

The typical presentation is an acute attack of pain, which often results in hospitalization. Recurrent acute attacks of pain eventually merge into chronic pancreatitis, with continuous pain and ultimately a steady loss of pancreatic function.

The median age at presentation is around 12 years, but presentation is earlier in children with an R122H mutation (10 years) than other patients (15 years), as shown in Figure 6.5. Most patients present by the age of 20 years and 95% by the age of 50 years. In the absence of a family history, the diagnosis of hereditary pancreatitis is commonly missed. Typically, children are thought to have a virus infection, Crohn's disease or psychosomatic pain (periodic syndrome). Young adults with hereditary or idiopathic chronic pancreatitis may be diagnosed with celiac disease or irritable bowel syndrome.

The median age for presentation for early-onset idiopathic chronic pancreatitis is 20–30 years, 35–45 years for alcoholic chronic pancreatitis, and 60 years for late-onset idiopathic chronic pancreatitis.

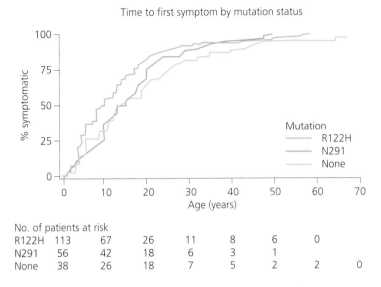

Time to first symptom by mutation status

No. of patients at risk							
R122H	113	67	26	11	8	6	0
N291	56	42	18	6	3	1	
None	38	26	18	7	5	2	2	0

Figure 6.5 Cumulative incidence of symptomatic presentation as abdominal pain in hereditary pancreatitis according to *PRSS1* mutation status: R122H or N29I mutations or no mutation. The data below the *x* axis indicate the number of patients at risk. Adapted from Howes et al. 2004.

Diagnosis and genetic testing

The diagnosis, as with all other types of chronic pancreatitis, will depend on clinical presentation and a combination of function and radiological investigations. The distinction between hereditary pancreatitis and idiopathic chronic pancreatitis requires a careful family history. A typical family tree of a patient with hereditary pancreatitis is shown in Figure 6.6. The detection of a *PRSS1* mutation will clinch the diagnosis, but it must be remembered that about 20% of patients do not have a mutation of this gene.

It is vital that patients undergo appropriate genetic counseling before any genetic tests are undertaken. A positive genetic test may help in the future management of any symptomatic children. Patients with idiopathic chronic pancreatitis are at a high risk of having a *CFTR* mutation; this may have significant implications for people planning to have children, particularly in areas where there are many carriers of the mutated *CFTR* gene in the general population. This is because there

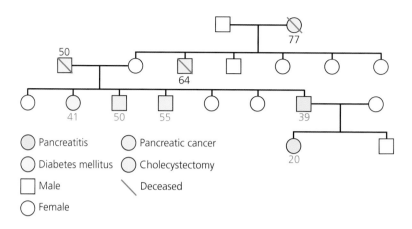

Figure 6.6 A typical family tree of a patient with hereditary pancreatitis.

will be an increased risk of parenting a child with cystic fibrosis – an autosomal-recessive condition caused by the inheritance of two mutated *CFTR* genes, one from each parent.

Management

The treatment of hereditary pancreatitis is at first identical to that of other forms of chronic pancreatitis. Alcohol consumption and tobacco smoking are both independent risk factors for chronic pancreatitis and pancreatic cancer and should therefore be strongly discouraged.

Genetic testing of symptomatic children of an individual with hereditary pancreatitis may be considered, together with appropriate genetic counseling, as this may help clinical diagnosis and management.

As with other forms of chronic pancreatitis, about 30% of patients will require active intervention by endoscopy and/or surgery because of local pancreatic complications or intractable pain. From the age of 40 years, patients with hereditary pancreatitis should be counseled regarding regular secondary screening for the detection of pancreatic cancer. International guidelines state that this should only take place at major regional pancreas centers. In appropriate cases, prophylactic total pancreatectomy may be offered – especially if there is complete endocrine and exocrine failure in conjunction with chronic abdominal pain that is difficult to control.

Future trends

- Routine genetic counseling and gene testing in regional pancreas centers for all families with hereditary and idiopathic pancreatitis
- Discovery of additional genes to explain nearly all cases of inherited pancreatitis
- New treatments to modify progression of the disease
- Improved methods of secondary screening to reduce deaths from pancreatic cancer.

Key points – hereditary pancreatitis

- Hereditary pancreatitis is an autosomal disease mainly caused by *PRSS1* mutations with 80% penetrance.
- Children and young adults are often misdiagnosed with other gastrointestinal diseases.
- There is a high risk of diabetes and pancreas exocrine failure and a lifetime risk of pancreatic cancer of 35%.
- Patients should undergo genetic counseling prior to genetic testing, and from the age of 40 years patients should be offered secondary screening for cancer in a regional pancreas cancer center.
- Alcohol and tobacco consumption should be strongly discouraged.
- Patients with idiopathic chronic pancreatitis are likely to carry *CFTR* mutations in one or both genes (compound heterozygotes).

Key references

Cohn JA, Friedman KJ, Noone PG et al. Relation between mutations of the cystic fibrosis gene and idiopathic pancreatitis. *N Engl J Med* 1998;339:653–8.

Gorry MC, Gabbaizedeh D, Furey W et al. Mutations in the cationic trypsinogen gene are associated with recurrent acute and chronic pancreatitis. *Gastroenterology* 1997;113:1063–8.

Howes N, Lerch MM, Greenhalf W et al.; European Registry of Hereditary Pancreatitis and Pancreatic Cancer (EUROPAC). Clinical and genetic characteristics of hereditary pancreatitis in Europe. *Clin Gastroenterol Hepatol* 2004;2:252–61.

Lowenfels AB, Maisonneuve P, DiMagno EP et al. Hereditary pancreatitis and the risk of pancreatic cancer. International Hereditary Pancreatitis Study Group. *J Natl Cancer Inst* 1997;89:442–6.

Lowenfels AB, Maisonneuve P, Whitcomb DC et al. Cigarette smoking as a risk factor for pancreatic cancer in patients with hereditary pancreatitis. *JAMA* 2001;286:169–70.

Noone PG, Zhou Z, Silverman LM et al. Cystic fibrosis gene mutations and pancreatitis risk: relation to epithelial ion transport and trypsin inhibitor gene mutations. *Gastroenterology* 2001;121: 1310–19.

Pfützer RH, Barmada MM, Brunskill AP et al. SPINK1/PSTI polymorphisms act as disease modifiers in familial and idiopathic chronic pancreatitis. *Gastroenterology* 2000;119: 615–23.

Pfützer RH, Barmada MM, Threadgold J, Greenhalf W, Ellis I et al. The N34S mutation of SPINK1 (PSTI) is associated with a familial pattern of idiopathic chronic pancreatitis but does not cause the disease. *Gut* 2002;50:675–81.

Whitcomb DC, Gorry MC, Preston RA et al. Hereditary pancreatitis is caused by a mutation in the cationic trypsinogen gene. *Nature Genet* 1996;14:141–5.

Witt H, Luck W, Becker M. A signal peptide cleavage site mutation in the cationic trypsinogen gene is strongly associated with chronic pancreatitis. *Gastroenterology* 1999;117:7–10.

Witt H, Luck W, Hennies HC et al. Mutations in the gene encoding the serine protease inhibitor, Kazal type 1 are associated with chronic pancreatitis. *Nature Genet* 2000; 25:213–16.

Epidemiology and natural history

Most cases of acute pancreatitis can be explained by gallstones, alcohol consumption or idiopathic pancreatitis (Figure 7.1), although there are many other causes (Table 7.1). The incidence of acute pancreatitis varies from 20 to 120 per 100 000 in the general population and is increasing steadily as a result of the rising age of the population and increasing alcohol consumption. Unlike chronic pancreatitis, once the patient has recovered from an attack of acute pancreatitis, there is complete resolution of symptoms and a return to normal anatomy and physiology. However, further attacks are likely under two circumstances:

• the initiating cause has not been removed (gallstones, alcohol consumption, etc.)

• there has been major pancreatic necrosis, resulting in chronic pancreatitis or main pancreatic duct stricture.

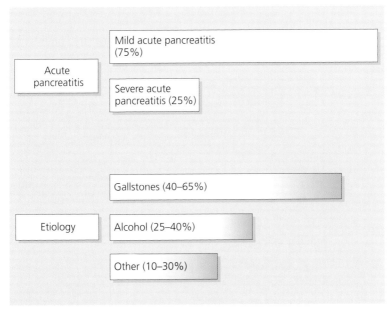

Figure 7.1 Epidemiology of acute pancreatitis.

TABLE 7.1

Causes of acute pancreatitis

Common causes

- Gallstones
- Alcohol consumption
- Idiopathic pancreatitis
- Pancreatic biopsy
- Endoscopic retrograde cholangiopancreato-graphy
- External trauma
- Intraoperative trauma
- Pancreatic cancer
- Ampullary cancer
- Pancreatic surgery
- Ischemia
- Postoperative (cardiac, renal and urological surgery)
- Hyperlipidemia
- Hypothermia

Less common causes

- Viral infection (mumps, human immunodeficiency virus)
- *Ascaris lumbricoides* (endemic areas)
- Scorpion bite (Trinidad and other endemic areas)
- Closed-loop duodenal obstruction
- Pancreatic stricture (postirradiation)
- Anti-acetylcholinesterase-containing insecticides
- Cobra venom
- Periampullary duodenal wall cysts
- Hypercalcemia – hyperparathyroidism
- Steroids
- Annular pancreas
- Hereditary pancreatitis
- Isolated autoimmune chronic pancreatitis
- Pancreatic divisum
- Sphincter of Oddi disorders (see Chapter 5, page 45)

The initial damage occurs in pancreatic acini subsequent to inappropriate trypsinogen activation. As well as autodigestion, the acini release chemokines that promote an extensive inflammatory cell infiltrate.

The disease quickly resolves in 75% of patients but in the other 25% the attack is severe. Mild disease is also called interstitial or edematous pancreatitis. Excessive stimulation of the white cells, coupled with the release of acute-phase proteins from the liver, results in a systemic inflammatory response syndrome (SIRS) (Figure 7.2).

Severe disease is defined by the Atlanta classification (Bradley 1993) as involving either a local or systemic complication. The development of complications follows a natural course, which can be divided into three overlapping phases (Figure 7.3). The SIRS is a feature of the first phase of acute pancreatitis and as such is not regarded as a complication but as a manifestation of the disease. However, a severe SIRS response will promote systemic complications that lead to multi-organ dysfunction syndrome (MODS).

Systemic complications

The likely systemic complications of acute pancreatitis include:

- respiratory failure, which may include unilateral or bilateral pleural effusions and may progress to full-blown adult respiratory distress syndrome
- renal failure
- central nervous system disturbances, including coma
- metabolic abnormalities – could include low arterial pH, low serum calcium and albumin and raised blood glucose and urea
- coagulation disorders – could include reduced clotting and abnormal platelet function, and may lead to disseminated intravascular coagulation with massive systemic bleeding
- MODS – more than one system may fail in the early phase (the first 2 weeks) of a severe attack; in the later phases multi-organ failure is usually secondary to sepsis from infected pancreatic necrosis.

Local complications

Pancreatic necrosis is accurately determined by contrast-enhanced computed tomography (CT). Necrosis may be observed early during an attack but often develops progressively. Initially the necrosis is not infected (sterile pancreatic necrosis). Pancreatic necrosis of less than 30% is rarely of clinical significance and is classed as mild pancreatitis.

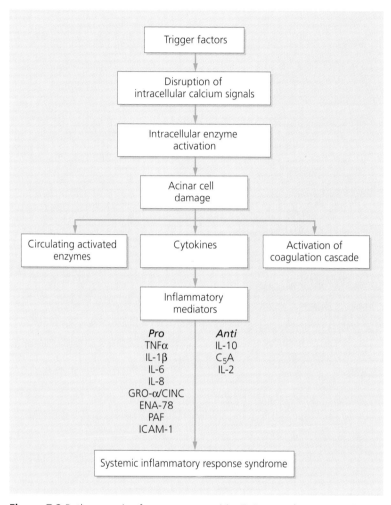

Figure 7.2 Pathogenesis of acute pancreatitis. C_5A, complement $_5A$; CINC, cytokine-induced neutrophil chemoattractant; ENA, epithelial neutrophil-activating [protein]; GRO, growth-related [protein]; ICAM, intercellular adhesion molecule; IL, interleukin; PAF, platelet-activating factor; TNFα, tumor necrosis factor α.

Acute fluid collections are common in acute pancreatitis, even in mild acute pancreatitis. They are not lined by either granulation (inflammatory) or fibrous tissue. The natural history is usually one of spontaneous resolution. Acute fluid collections that are rich in

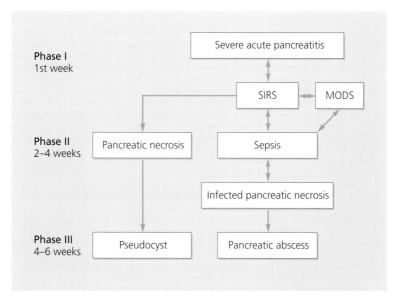

Figure 7.3 The three phases of acute pancreatitis. MODS, multi-organ dysfunction syndrome; SIRS, systemic inflammatory response syndrome.

pancreatic enzymes may progress to pancreatic pseudocysts (described below).

Infected pancreatic necrosis is a secondary infection of sterile pancreatic necrosis and develops in the later phase in 40–70% of patients with severe disease. By definition, it is retroperitoneal and commonly extends down the left and sometimes the right paracolic gutter surrounding the kidneys. The necrosis may extend into the pelvis or chest and occurs by spread of bacteria from the gastrointestinal tract, biliary tree or skin or by iatrogenic intervention. Gas-forming bacteria are commonly involved and gas within the area of infected pancreatic necrosis is a common late feature. The infected necrosis acts as a major focus of infection, leading to septicemia and amplification of SIRS and MODS. The overall mortality in this group of patients is 20–40%.

Secondary fungal infection is frequently associated with antibiotic treatment of infected pancreatic necrosis and significantly raises mortality.

Hepatic portal and/or splenic vein thrombosis is associated with protracted recovery from extensive pancreatic necrosis. The consequence is left-sided portal hypertension, with the development of venous collaterals and gastric varices.

Hemorrhage may occur from necrotizing pancreatitis and erosion of major vessels within or close to the pancreas.

Colonic necrosis may occur because of involvement of colonic vessels (commonly the middle colic and marginal arteries), leading to colonic necrosis and fecal peritonitis.

Pancreatic fistula. A fistula is usually an abnormal communication between two epithelial surfaces, but the term is also used if there is an abnormal communication between a hollow viscus, such as the colon or duodenum, and the area of pancreatic necrosis. This will lead to gas within the area of pancreatic necrosis.

Pancreatic pseudocysts are rich in pancreatic enzymes and lined by granulation (inflammatory) and fibrous tissue. By definition, a pseudocyst will not be properly formed for at least 4 weeks from the start of an attack. Most pseudocysts resolve spontaneously.

Pancreatic abscess is a localized collection of pus and occurs in the final phase of acute pancreatitis. In contrast to infected pancreatic necrosis, the mortality is only 5–10%.

Clinical presentation

The initial presentation of both mild and acute pancreatitis is similar. There is a sudden and severe onset of epigastric pain that may remain in the epigastrium or spread into the central back and the whole of the abdomen. The patient may be unable to move because of the pain, refuses food and water and may vomit. These symptoms are accompanied by the SIRS, which comprises two or more of the following:

- temperature above 38°C or below 36°C
- heart rate above 90 beats/minute

- respiratory rate greater than 20 breaths/minute or $PaCO_2$ below 4.3 kPa
- white cell count above 12×10^9 cells/L or below 4×10^9 cells/L, or more than 10% immature cells.

   Common symptoms and signs (Table 7.2) may be confused with those of a number of acute conditions above or below the diaphragm:

- perforated peptic ulcer
- leaking aortic aneurysm
- mesenteric infarction
- myocardial infarction
- perforated esophagus
- gastroesophageal reflux
- pneumonia
- acute cholecystitis
- biliary colic
- peptic ulcer disease.

Diagnosis

The diagnosis is based on a typical clinical presentation plus a serum amylase that is three times the upper of limit of normal within 2–3 days of the onset of symptoms. The serum amylase peaks at about 24 hours after the onset of the attack and then declines exponentially over the next 5–7 days. Thus, if the amylase is measured at day 4 or 5 after the onset of the attack, it may be only marginally raised or within normal limits. Urinary amylase may be cleared more slowly, but the diagnostic threshold is much higher (tenfold). Absence of gas on an erect plain abdominal and chest radiograph will eliminate most large gastrointestinal perforations. *If there is any doubt about the diagnosis, an emergency contrast-enhanced CT scan must be performed.*

Medical treatment

The principles are basic resuscitation and close monitoring in an appropriate setting, ranging from an acute admissions ward to an intensive therapy unit. The essential requirements are as follows:

- 1–4 hourly monitoring of pulse, blood pressure, temperature and urine output

TABLE 7.2

Symptoms and signs of acute pancreatitis

Common findings

- Abdominal pain
- Nausea and vomiting
- Abdominal tenderness
- Paralytic ileus
- Fever
- Abdominal distension
- Tachycardia
- Tachypnea
- Jaundice
- Respiratory insufficiency
- Hypovolemia
- Shock
- Pleural effusion
- Cardiac insufficiency
- Renal insufficiency

Less common findings

- Ascites
- Symptomatic hypocalcemia
- Massive intra-abdominal hemorrhage
- Disseminated intravascular coagulation
- Subcutaneous fat necrosis
- Hepatic portal vein thrombosis
- Periumbilical darkening of the skin (from blood) – Cullen's sign
- Local areas of discoloration in the region of the loins (due to retroperitoneal hemorrhage) – Grey Turner's sign
- Infra-inguinal bruising – Fox's sign
- Pericardial effusion
- Cardiac tamponade
- Hematemesis
- Melena
- Polyarthritis
- Bone marrow fat necrosis
- Focal cerebral necrosis
- Encephalopathy
- Sudden blindness

- baseline chest radiograph and measurement of arterial blood gases
- complete blood count and measurement of basic electrolytes, albumin, proteins, liver enzymes, bilirubin, calcium, glucose, urea and C-reactive protein (CRP).

Predicting severity. It is important to determine as early as possible whether the attack of pancreatitis is likely to be mild or severe. Clinical judgement can be difficult, especially during the first 24–48 hours when the severity of disease may change rapidly. One or more of the following methods may be used; they are all of similar accuracy in predicting outcome.

CT scanning is used to help establish the diagnosis in uncertain cases and to assist in determining the need for and extent of surgical intervention (pancreatic necrosectomy, colectomy for necrosis, etc.).

Serum CRP. A serum CRP level above 150 mg/L indicates a severe attack, but the peak is not reached until 72 hours after symptom onset (Figure 7.4).

Clinicobiochemical criteria. The Ranson score includes 11 criteria variously applicable at 24 and 48 hours and separate systems for alcohol- and gallstone-associated acute pancreatitis. The Imrie or Glasgow system is much simpler, requiring only eight criteria at 48 hours, and is just as accurate (Table 7.3).

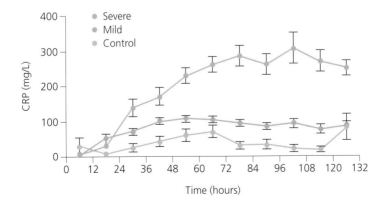

Figure 7.4 Time course of serum C-reactive protein (CRP) in acute pancreatitis from symptom onset. Adapted from Neoptolemos et al. 2000.

TABLE 7.3

Glasgow or Imrie criteria – simplified Ranson criteria for predicting the severity of an attack of acute pancreatitis

The mnemonic 'PANCREAS' makes this easy to remember.

P   Arterial PaO_2 < 9 kPa

A   Albumin < 32 g/L

N   Urea nitrogen >10 mmol/L

C   Calcium < 2 mmol/L

R   Raised white cell count: > 16 mmol/L

E   Enzyme: lactate dehydrogenase > 600 mmol/L

A   Age > 55 years

S   Sugar: glucose >10 mmol/L

The presence of three or more criteria reached before or at 48 hours of an attack predicts a severe attack; two or fewer predicts a mild attack. The maximum sensitivity for a severe attack and the maximum specificity for a mild attack are achieved at 48 hours after the start of an attack.

APACHE II score (Acute Physiology And Chronic Health Evaluation) can be applied at any time but is cumbersome, requiring 15 different clinical and biochemical criteria (Figure 7.5).

Balthazar CT score is based on the extent of pancreatic necrosis and the number of acute fluid collections.

Severe acute pancreatitis. Patients with a severe attack will need to be managed on an intensive therapy unit and may require two or more of the following:

- continuous arterial and central venous pressure monitoring
- intubation for assisted respiratory ventilation
- inotropes for cardiac support
- hemofiltration or hemodialysis for renal failure
- nutrition by a nasojejunal tube to provide early enteral nutrition (additional parenteral nutrition may also be required for sufficient calories).

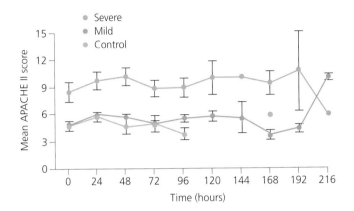

Figure 7.5 Time course of the APACHE II (Acute Physiology And Chronic Health Evaluation) scores in severe acute pancreatitis from symptom onset. Adapted from Neoptolemos et al. 2000.

Overviews of the management for mild and severe attacks are given in Figures 7.6 and 7.7, respectively.

Endoscopic treatment. Endoscopic retrograde cholangio-pancreatography (ERCP) with a view to endoscopic sphincterotomy is required as follows.

- In patients with a predicted severe attack of acute pancreatitis secondary to gallstones, ERCP will reduce morbidity and mortality from acute pancreatitis. The presence of gallbladder stones is often missed by abdominal ultrasound during an acute attack. An elevated serum alanine transaminase level (> 60 iu/L) within 48 hours of an attack is just as accurate as ultrasound, if not more so.
- For main bile duct stones found by intraoperative cholangiography, routine cholangiography during laparoscopic cholecystectomy followed by selective postoperative endoscopic sphincterotomy has been found to be more efficient than routine preoperative ERCP.
- ERCP can be used to prevent further attacks in patients who are not fit enough to undergo laparoscopic cholecystectomy.

A cholecystectomy or endoscopic sphincterotomy should be performed in all patients before discharge from hospital, as they

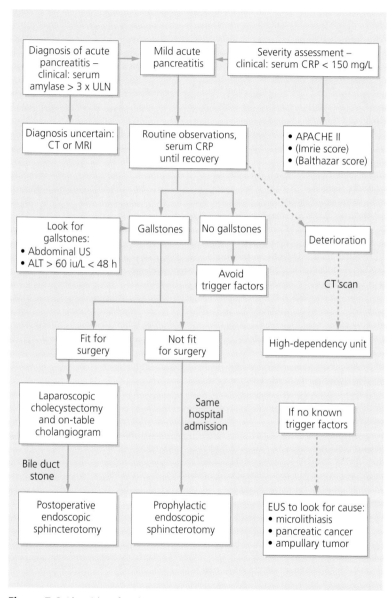

Figure 7.6 Algorithm for the management of mild acute pancreatitis. ALT, alanine aminotransferase; APACHE, Acute Physiology And Chronic Health Evaluation; CRP, C-reactive protein; CT, computed tomography; EUS, endoscopic ultrasound; MRI, magnetic resonance imaging; ULN, upper limit of normal; US, ultrasonography.

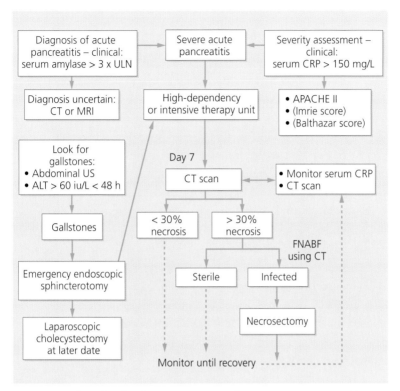

Figure 7.7 Algorithm for the management of severe acute pancreatitis. ALT, alanine aminotransferase; APACHE, Acute Physiology And Chronic Health Evaluation; CRP, C-reactive protein; CT, computed tomography; FNABF, fine-needle aspiration for bacteriology and fungi; MRI, magnetic resonance imaging; ULN, upper limit of normal; US, ultrasonography.

run a high risk of recurrent attacks of acute pancreatitis, along with the attendant morbidity and mortality.

Surgical treatment

The principal purpose of surgery in severe acute pancreatitis is the removal of dead pancreatic tissue. The indications are:

- infected pancreatic necrosis (absolute indication)
- extensive sterile pancreatic necrosis, with no improvement of symptoms following at least two weeks of optimal care from the detection of extensive necrosis (relative indication).

Because the features of the SIRS are identical to those of sepsis (defined as SIRS with proven infection), clinical parameters may not identify pancreatic infection before it is too late. Thus, from day 7 of a severe attack, all patients must undergo a contrast-enhanced CT scan, repeated at 7–10-day intervals until there are signs of clinical improvement. If there is necrosis, there should be weekly CT-guided fine-needle aspiration for bacteriology and fungi. If this becomes positive, surgical intervention is mandatory. Three main techniques can be used for necrosectomy:

- open necrosectomy with closed lesser sac lavage
- repeated laparotomies with zipper to close the peritoneum after each intervention or left open as laparostomy
- minimally invasive necrosectomy – the videoscopic retroperitoneal approach has the best results.

Many drugs have been used in an attempt to modify the severity of an attack of acute pancreatitis (such as trasylol, octreotide and lexipafant) as well as prophylactic antibiotics to prevent the development of infected pancreatic necrosis, but none has been shown conclusively to be effective.

Follow-up

In order to prevent further attacks, known trigger factors of the attack should be avoided (for example alcohol, if that was the cause). If there is no known trigger factor then endoscopic ultrasound should be used to look for a cause – particularly microlithiasis (small gallstones), pancreatic cancer or ampullary tumor.

There are no long-term sequelae following recovery from mild acute pancreatitis. In severe necrotizing pancreatitis, however, there are significant late complications in up to 60% of patients. These include:

- delayed collections
- pancreatic exocrine insufficiency
- diabetes mellitus
- pancreatic pseudocyst
- biliary stricture.

Thus, long-term follow-up is required to monitor the development of these complications.

Future trends

- Early prognostication using one or two rapid blood tests
- More extensive use of emergency endoscopic sphincterotomy for bile duct stones in severe disease
- Improved and earlier detection of infected pancreatic necrosis
- Better results from minimally invasive pancreatic necrosectomy
- Drugs that will modify the progression of mild-to-severe acute pancreatitis
- More effective measures to treat the excessive systemic inflammatory response syndrome and prevent multi-organ dysfunction
- Better treatment of multi-organ failure.

Key points – acute pancreatitis

- Undertake a contrast-enhanced CT scan if there is any doubt about the diagnosis of acute pancreatitis.
- Prognostic evaluation for the severity of the disease within the first 3 days of symptom onset.
- Determine whether gallstones are the cause of the attack and, if so, ensure urgent endoscopic sphincterotomy; mild cases need to have cholecystectomy or, if not fit for surgery, endoscopic sphincterotomy to prevent further attacks.
- If severe with extensive necrosis beyond the first week, undertake fine-needle aspiration for bacteriology and fungi; if there is proven infected necrosis, pancreatic necrosectomy is required.
- If the etiology is uncertain, undertake endoscopic ultrasonography following resolution of the attack to exclude unusual mechanical causes such as a small tumor.

Key references

Balthazar E. Acute pancreatitis: assessment of severity with clinical and CT evaluation. *Radiology* 2002;223:603–13.

Beger HG, Bittner R, Block S, Büchler M. Bacterial contamination of pancreatic necrosis. *Gastroenterology* 1986;91:433–8.

Beger HG, Büchler M, Bittner R et al. Necrosectomy and postoperative local lavage in necrotizing pancreatitis. *Br J Surg* 1988;75:207–12.

Bradley III E. A clinically based classification system for acute pancreatitis. *Arch Surg* 1993;128: 586–90.

Connor S, Alexakis N, Neal T et al. Fungal infection but not type of bacterial infection is associated with a high mortality in primary and secondary infected pancreatic necrosis. *Dig Surg* 2004;21:297–304.

Connor S, Ghaneh P, Raraty M et al. Increasing age and APACHE II scores are the main determinants of outcome following pancreatic necrosectomy. *Br J Surg* 2003; 90:1542–8.

Dellinger R, Carlet J, Masur H et al. Surviving sepsis. Campaign guidelines for management of severe sepsis and septic shock. *Crit Care Med* 2004;32:858–73.

Isenmann R, Rau B, Beger HG. Bacterial infection and extent of necrosis are determinants of organ failure in patients with acute necrotizing pancreatitis. *Br J Surg* 1999;86:1020–4.

Isenmann R, Runzi M, Kron M et al. Prophylactic antibiotic treatment in patients with predicted severe acute pancreatitis: A placebo-controlled, double-blind trial. *Gastroenterology* 2004;126:997–1004.

Marik PE, Zaloga GP. Meta-analysis of parenteral nutrition versus enteral nutrition in patients with acute pancreatitis. *BMJ* 2004;328: 1407–23.

Neoptolemos JP, Carr-Locke DL, London NJ et al. Controlled trial of urgent endoscopic retrograde cholangiopancreatography and endoscopic sphincterotomy versus conservative treatment for acute pancreatitis due to gallstones. *Lancet* 1988;2:979–83.

Neoptolemos J, Kemppainen E, Mayer J et al. Early prediction of severity in acute pancreatitis by urinary trypsinogen activation peptide: a multicentre study. *Lancet* 2000;355:1955–60.

Raraty M, Ward J, Erdemli G et al. Calcium-dependent enzyme activation and vacuole formation in the apical granular region of pancreatic acinar cells. *Proc Natl Acad Sci USA* 2000;97:13 126–31.

Uhl W, Warshaw A, Imrie C et al. IAP guidelines for the surgical management of acute pancreatitis. *Pancreatology* 2002;2:565–73.

Epidemiology and pathology

Chronic pancreatitis is a progressive inflammatory process of the pancreas that leads to irreversible destruction of the pancreas.

The prevalence of chronic pancreatitis varies enormously, from 20 to 200 per 100 000 in the general population, and is increasing as a result of environmental factors and in particular the rising consumption of alcohol. Genetic factors also contribute to the development of chronic pancreatitis (Table 8.1). Approximately 70% of cases are associated with alcohol consumption, and tobacco smoking is an independent risk

TABLE 8.1

Classification of chronic pancreatitis and risk factors

Toxic–metabolic pancreatitis

- Alcohol consumption
- Tobacco smoking
- Hypocalcemia – hyperparathyroidism
- Chronic renal failure
- Medications
- Phenacetin abuse (possibly from chronic renal insufficiency)
- Toxins
- Organotin compounds (e.g. di-*n*-butyltin dichloride)

Idiopathic pancreatitis

- Early onset
- Late onset
- Tropical
- Tropical calcific pancreatitis
- Fibrocalculous pancreatic diabetes

(CONTINUED)

TABLE 8.1 (CONTINUED)

Classification of chronic pancreatitis and risk factors

Genetic pancreatitis
- Autosomal-dominant – mutations in the *PRSS1* gene (also known as the *cationic trypsinogen* gene)
- Autosomal-recessive and modifier genes
  - *CFTR* mutations
  - *SPINK1* mutations

Autoimmune pancreatitis
- Isolated autoimmune chronic pancreatitis
- Syndromic autoimmune chronic pancreatitis
  - Chronic pancreatitis associated with Sjögren's syndrome
  - Chronic pancreatitis associated with inflammatory bowel disease
  - Chronic pancreatitis associated with primary biliary cirrhosis

Recurrent and severe acute pancreatitis
- Postnecrotic (severe acute pancreatitis)
- Recurrent acute pancreatitis
- Vascular diseases/ischemia
- Postirradiation

Obstructive pancreatitis
- Pancreatic divisum
- Sphincter of Oddi disorders (see Chapter 5, page 45)
- Duct obstruction (e.g. by tumor)
- Periampullary duodenal wall cysts
- Post-traumatic pancreatic duct scars

CFTR, cystic fibrosis transmembrane conductance regulator (gene); *PRSS1, protease serine 1* (gene); *SPINK1, serine protease inhibitor, kazal type 1* (gene).

factor. About 25% of the remaining cases are classed as idiopathic but a high proportion of these have mutations of the *CFTR* (*cystic fibrosis transmembrane conductance regulator*) gene and the *SPINK1* (*pancreatic secretory trypsin inhibitor*) gene.

The pathological features of chronic pancreatitis are:

- disruption of the lobular parenchymal architecture, with extensive destruction of pancreatic acini (and subsequently islets of Langerhans) and replacement by fibrous or fatty tissue
- chronic inflammatory infiltrate
- pancreatic ductal and parenchymal calcification.

Once initiated, the disease follows a relentless course. The primary injury appears to occur in the acinar cells but injury to the pancreatic ducts may also be contributory. In consequence of this injury, the stellate cells are stimulated to produce excessive amounts of fibrous tissues (Figure 8.1). As the disease progresses, chronic inflammation not only

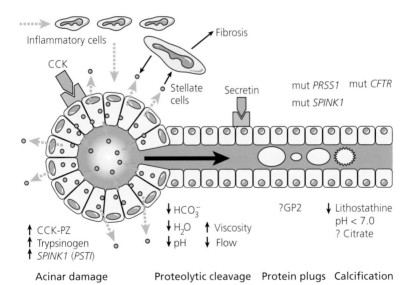

Figure 8.1 Schematic representation of the pathophysiology of chronic pancreatitis. CCK, cholecystokinin; PZ, pancreozymin; *CFTR, cystic fibrosis transmembrane conductance regulator* gene; GP2, G-protein 2; HCO_3^-, bicarbonate; *PRSS1, protease serine 1* (gene); *SPINK1 (PST1), serine protease inhibitor, kazal type 1* (*pancreatic secretory trypsin inhibitor*) gene.

destroys the gland itself but has major effects on surrounding structures, with serious consequences (Table 8.2). Elimination of environmental

TABLE 8.2

Complications of chronic pancreatitis

- Pancreatic exocrine deficiency, leading to severe weight loss
- Pancreatic endocrine insufficiency, leading to diabetes mellitus requiring insulin therapy
- Pain
- Pseudocyst
- Stricture of the main pancreatic duct
- Main pancreatic duct stones
- Parenchymal stones
- Biliary obstruction
- Duodenal obstruction
- Pancreatic ascites – free pancreatic juice in the abdominal cavity secondary to disruption of the main pancreatic duct or a communicating pseudocyst
- Pancreatic fistula – a communication between the main pancreatic duct and an internal organ (such as the peritoneal cavity) or the skin (external fistula)
- Hepatic portal venous compression or occlusion
- Sinistral portal hypertension – selective increased venous pressure in the left side of the hepatic portal system
- Gastric varices
- Pseudo-aneurysm, commonly caused by erosion of a pseudocyst into a major visceral vessel (such as the splenic artery)
- Pancreatic ductal adenocarcinoma (20-fold risk or 5% of all patients)
- Social and professional disruption

risk factors such as alcohol consumption and tobacco smoking may modify the long-term outcome.

Causes of pain in chronic pancreatitis

The pain of chronic pancreatitis is multifactorial in origin, but modern theories principally relate to nerve alterations (Figure 8.2).

- The number and diameter of intra- and interlobular nerve bundles in pancreatic tissue is increased.
- The perineurium is damaged – GAP-43 (growth-associated protein 43, a marker of neural plasticity) is significantly increased in pancreatic nerve fibers.
- Levels of neurotransmitters such as calcitonin gene-related peptide and substance P are increased.
- Inflammatory cells interact with the damaged nerves (neuroimmune interactions). Expression of nerve growth factor and tyrosine kinase receptor A is increased and has a significant relationship with pain intensity.

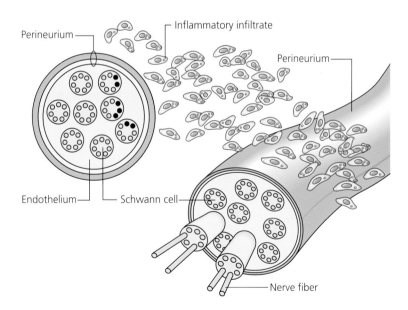

Figure 8.2 The pain of chronic pancreatitis may be caused by disruption of the perineurium and inflammatory infiltrate.

- Pain may be increased as a consequence of local complications such as pseudocysts and biliary tract or duodenal obstruction.
- Pain is also associated with inability to digest fat properly – malabsorption.
- Older theories include increased intraductal pressure and compartment syndrome.

Clinical presentation

About 80% of patients with chronic pancreatitis experience pain, and about 50% develop pancreatic exocrine and endocrine deficiency some 20 years after disease onset. Pancreatic exocrine insufficiency occurs when there is destruction of more than 90% of the parenchyma and manifests as steatorrhea (Figure 8.3).

Features of pancreatic exocrine failure include:
- weight loss
- steatorrhea – fatty stool: more than 7 g fat excreted per day on a normal fat diet

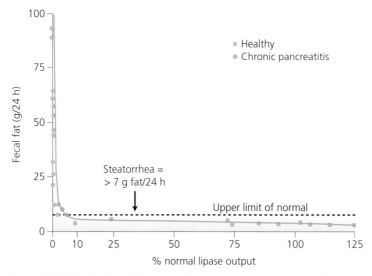

Figure 8.3 Relationship of fat excretion to pancreatic exocrine function measured as a proportion of normal lipase output. From DiMagno et al. 1973. Copyright © 1973 Massachusetts Medical Society. All rights reserved.

- avoidance of fat
- vitamin deficiency
- abdominal pain
- peptic ulcer: caused by loss of bicarbonate secretion (normally produced by the pancreatic ductal cells) and thus loss of buffering capacity against gastric acid arriving in the duodenum from the stomach.

Features of pancreatic endocrine failure include:
- weight loss
- polydypsia
- polyuria
- diabetic ketoacidosis and coma.

Complications of pancreatitis include:
- abdominal pain (intermittent or continuous, with increased pain during exacerbations); typically the pain is in the epigastrium and the back, and is relieved by flexion
- abdominal mass – pseudocyst or pancreatic cancer
- jaundice due to biliary obstruction
- vomiting due to duodenal obstruction
- abdominal distension due to pancreatic ascites
- upper gastrointestinal hemorrhage due to gastric varices
- massive intra-abdominal bleeding due to pseudo-aneurysm
- cachexia secondary to pancreatic ductal adenocarcinoma.

Typically patients have lost the support of their friends and family or their employment, especially if the pancreatitis is associated with alcohol consumption.

Diagnosis

The diagnosis will depend on clinical presentation and a combination of functional and radiological investigations, although the latter may appear entirely normal even in late-stage disease.

Blood tests. The amylase level may be elevated during an acute exacerbation. Liver tests may indicate biochemical biliary obstruction. Autoantibodies indicate autoimmune chronic pancreatitis.

Fecal elastase is a simple test and is useful if the result is clearly abnormal (< 200 µg/g).

Pancreatolauryl test is a more accurate determinant than fecal elastase, but requires a 3-day complete urine collection.

Secretin test is the best of the functional tests but is performed only in specialist centers as it requires intubation of the stomach and duodenum and continuous aspiration of pancreatic secretions for 2 hours after stimulation by intravenous secretin.

Plain abdominal radiography may show calcification of the pancreas.

Endoscopic ultrasonography (EUS) is a highly sensitive test for chronic pancreatitis in moderate to severe form; a normal EUS correlates well with the absence of chronic pancreatitis. Because of the high sensitivity, minimal or early changes of chronic pancreatitis should be interpreted with caution; overdiagnosis is possible, as there is overlap with age-related changes, and there are more issues with interobserver variability in the case of minimal or equivocal changes.

Contrast-enhanced computed tomography (CT) may show ductal abnormalities, pseudocyst or vascular complications. A pancreatic pseudocyst should be be differentiated from a pancreatic cystic cancer. CT is very sensitive at detecting calcification; both solid and cystic tumors of the pancreas can be calcified.

Magnetic resonance cholangiopancreatography (MRCP) may reveal abnormalities in the biliary and pancreatic ducts, such as strictures and dilation.

Tissue diagnosis by EUS. EUS-guided fine-needle aspiration or the recently developed EUS-guided Trucut biopsy technique appear as attractive options for cytological or tissue diagnosis of chronic pancreatitis. However, the application of these techniques for chronic pancreatitis is still developing (along with concern about complications, especially with EUS-guided Trucut biopsy) and they are not yet used routinely.

Positron-emission tomography may not reliably distinguish chronic pancreatitis from pancreatic cancer.

Medical treatment

Elimination of environmental risk factors such as alcohol consumption and tobacco smoking may modify symptoms and, to some extent, the long-term outcome. Before any type of interventional treatment is considered, medical management must be optimized. The factors governing appropriate fat digestion are complex (Figure 8.4). Fat intake should not be restricted but sufficient pancreatic enzyme supplementation with each meal must be ensured. Replacement of lipase is the key factor – up to 800 000 units, divided between meals, may be necessary every day. The addition of a proton-pump inhibitor is of particular importance, as this will increase duodenal pH and improve lipase activity.

Other medical treatments include:
- treatment of diabetes
- analgesia
- psychosocial support.

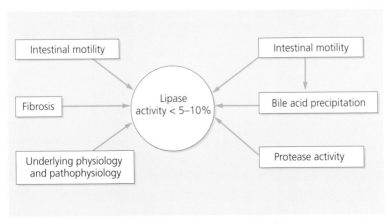

Figure 8.4 Factors affecting pancreatic lipase activity following pancreatic resection.

Patients with intermittent pain appear to have a more favorable disease course.

The American Gastroenterological Association has produced guidelines for the management of pain, which can be quite problematic (Figure 8.5). Family and psychosocial support is particularly important. For patients with an alcohol problem it is important that any employment involving alcohol (such as the entertainment industry) should be changed.

Endoscopic treatment

Relieving main pancreatic duct obstruction caused by stones and/or strictures requires the use of stents and extracorporeal shock-wave lithotripsy but is only applicable to simple structures and single duct stones. There is little effect on pain and it does not influence the development of pancreatic insufficiency.

Drainage of the biliary tree. Endoscopic stenting may be used as a temporary measure, but the medium- and long-term success rate is poor.

Drainage of pancreatic pseudocysts. Many pseudocysts resolve spontaneously (Table 8.3); only persisting, symptomatic pseudocysts require treatment. Pseudocysts may be drained into the stomach or duodenum using a transmural or transpapillary technique. The morbidity is 15% (mortality 0.25%) with a technical success rate of 20%. The long-term recurrence rate is about 12%. Relatively simple pseudocysts without parenchymal disease are most suitable for endoscopic treatment.

Celiac plexus block under EUS guidance or percutaneous routes may be undertaken in some patients, but generally one should not expect long-term pain relief. Limited data comparing the two techniques suggest that EUS-guided route may be more effective. Most clinicians prefer to do a block with steroids and bupivacaine instead of using ablative or sclerosing agents like alcohol in chronic pancreatitis, because of the higher risk of irreversible complications (e.g neurological), and because

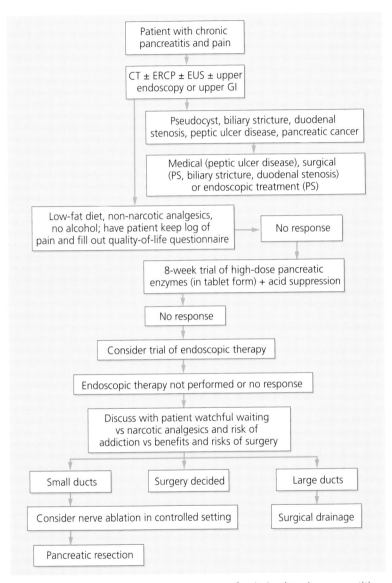

Figure 8.5 Guidelines for the management of pain in chronic pancreatitis developed by the American Gastroenterological Association. BS, biliary stricture; CT, computed tomography; DS, duodenal stenosis; ERCP, endoscopic retrograde cholangiopancreatography; EUS, endoscopic ultrasound; GI, gastrointestinal; PS, pancreatic duct stricture. Adapted from American Gastroenterological Association, 1998.

TABLE 8.3

Factors associated with pseudocyst resolution

- Acute pancreatitis
- Small pseudocysts
- Intrapancreatic pseudocyst
- Pseudocyst of the head of the pancreas
- Persistence < 6 weeks
- Thin pseudocyst wall

any subsequent surgery may also be difficult owing to intense fibrosis around major vessels.

Surgical treatment

Bilateral thoracoscopic splanchnicectomy is a minimally invasive thoracic approach that divides the greater, lesser and least splanchnic nerves of the sympathetic system, which carry afferent pain fibers from the pancreas. This procedure provides good short-term pain relief in about 50% of patients – particularly those with no prior intervention – but the benefit is greatly reduced in the long term.

Pancreatic duct drainage procedures. Lateral pancreatojejunostomy requires a dilated duct of at least 6–7 mm diameter and is associated with a low mortality (up to 5%) and morbidity. Pain relief is good to moderate in 80% of patients in the short-term but only 50–60% of patients are pain-free at 5 years. There is little effect on pain in patients with advanced chronic pancreatitis.

Drainage of pancreatic pseudocysts. The indications for surgical internal drainage of pancreatic pseudocysts include:
- contraindication or failure of endoscopic and radiological methods
- associated complex pathology, such as an inflammatory mass in the head of the pancreas
- pseudocysts with complex or multiple main pancreatic duct strictures

- pseudocysts with a main bile duct stricture
- venous occlusive disease
- multiple pseudocysts
- most pseudocysts of the pancreatic tail.

The techniques include pseudocystjejunostomy, pseudocystgastrostomy and pseudocystduodenostomy and have a 95–100% success rate, with a long-term recurrence rate of 5%. The operative morbidity is 15%, with a mortality rate of 1–3%, depending on the complexity of the underlying disease.

Bypass of biliary or duodenal obstruction. Biliary stricture occurs in 6% of patients and duodenal obstruction in 1%. Choledocho-jejunostomy or choledochoduodenostomy are performed for bile duct stricture, and gastrojejunostomy for duodenal obstruction. The success rates are over 98%. Combined obstruction of the pancreatic duct, main bile duct and duodenum requires a resection, or double drainage if this is not possible.

Pancreatic resection achieves the best results for intractable pain in chronic pancreatitis. Long-term pain relief is achieved in 70–95% of patients, but there is a still a mortality of 1–3%. The outcome is better if patients have not been long-term heavy users of opioid analgesia (Figure 8.6).

Pylorus-preserving Kausch–Whipple partial pancreatoduodenectomy is still valuable if the pancreatic parenchyma is relatively 'soft'.

Beger operation – resection of the head of the pancreas preserving the duodenum – is appropriate for a dominant inflammatory mass in the head of the pancreas or small duct disease (Figure 8.7).

Frey procedure combines lateral pancreatojejunostomy with removal of some of the tissue in the head of the pancreas.

Left ('distal') pancreatectomy with spleen preservation is used for dominant left-sided disease.

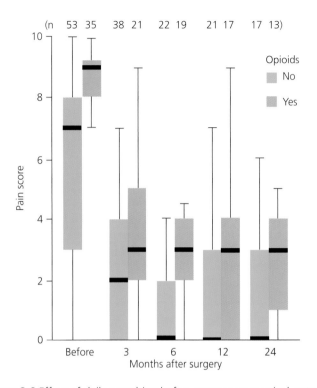

Figure 8.6 Effect of daily morphine before surgery on surgical outcome. The vertical axis shows preoperative pain scores (visual analog scale 0–10). Box plots show the median (bar), interquartile range and extremes within each group. n = number of patients at risk at each time point. Adapted from Alexakis et al. 2004.

Total pancreatectomy with preservation of the duodenum and spleen is indicated for patients with disabling pain for whom previous partial resection has failed or for those with total endocrine and exocrine pancreatic failure. The operation is also indicated as prophylaxis against cancer in hereditary pancreatitis.

Future trends
• Earlier referral to pancreas treatment centers
• Genetic counseling and intervention in patients with hereditary and idiopathic chronic pancreatitis

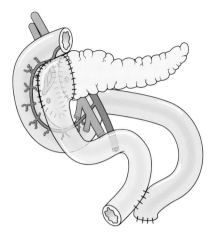

Figure 8.7 Beger operation – duodenum-preserving resection of the head of the pancreas.

- Drugs that will modify the progression of the disease
- Genetically engineered insulin-producing cells
- Effective secondary screening for pancreatic cancer
- More effective pain control measures
- Further refinement of surgical techniques.

Key points – chronic pancreatitis

- The diagnosis must be clearly established by radiological and/or functional tests.
- Risk factors such as smoking and alcohol should be discouraged.
- Medical measures should be optimized.
- Severe pain needs specialist surgical referral before daily use of powerful opiates becomes established.
- Pancreatic cancer may develop within the chronic pancreatitis.

Key references

Adamek H, Jakobs R, Buttmann A et al. Long term follow up of patients with chronic pancreatitis and pancreatic stones treated with extracorporeal shock wave lithotripsy. *Gut* 1999;45:402–5.

Alexakis N, Connor S, Ghaneh P et al. Influence of opioid use on surgical and long term outcome following resection for chronic pancreatitis. *Surgery* 2004;136:600–8.

American Gastroenterological Association medical position statement: treatment of pain in chronic pancreatitis. *Gastroenterology* 1998;115:763–4.

Ammann R, Akovbiantz A, Largiader F, Schueler G. Course and outcome of chronic pancreatitis. Longitudinal study of a mixed medical-surgical series of 245 patients. *Gastroenterology* 1984;86:820–8.

Beger H, Schlosser W, Friess H, Büchler M. Duodenum-preserving head resection in chronic pancreatitis changes the natural course of the disease. *Ann Surg* 1999;230:512–23.

Bockman D, Büchler M, Malfertheiner P, Beger H. Analysis of nerves in chronic pancreatitis. *Gastroenterology* 1988;94:1459–69.

DiMagno E. Towards understanding (and management) of painful chronic pancreatitis. *Gastroenterology* 1999;116:1252–7.

DiMagno EP, Go VL, Summerskill WH. Relations between pancreatic enzyme ouputs and malabsorption in severe pancreatic insufficiency. *N Engl J Med* 1973;288:813–15.

Etemad B, Whitcomb D. Chronic pancreatitis: Diagnosis, classification and new genetic developments. *Gastroenterology* 2001;120: 682–707.

Friess H, Shrikhande M, Martignoni M et al. Neural alterations in surgical stage chronic pancreatitis are independent of the underlying aetiology. *Gut* 2002;50:682–6.

Layer P, Yamamoto H, Kalthoff L et al. The different courses of early- and late-onset idiopathic and alcoholic chronic pancreatitis. *Gastroenterology* 1994;107:1481–7.

Lowenfels A, Maisonneuve P, Cavallini G et al. Pancreatitis and the risk of pancreatic cancer. *N Engl J Med* 1993;328:1433–7.

Tinto A, Lloyd D, Kang J et al. Acute and chronic pancreatitis – diseases on the rise: a study of hospital admissions in England 1989/90–1999/2000. *Aliment Pharmacol Ther* 2002;16:2097–105.

Warshaw A, Banks P, Fernandez-Del Castillo P. AGA technical review: Treatment of pain in chronic pancreatitis. *Gastroenterology* 1998;115:765–76.

Epidemiology and pathology

The term pancreatic cancer usually refers to the common pancreatic ductal adenocarcinoma, although there is a large variety of other exocrine tumor types (Table 9.1), with varying prognoses.

Pancreatic cancer usually arises in the head of the pancreas (80%) and less commonly in the body (15%) and tail (5%). Tumors arising in the pancreas or in close proximity to it include:

TABLE 9.1

Common exocrine epithelial tumors of the pancreas

Benign tumors
- Serous cystadenoma
- Hamartoma

Borderline tumors
- Intraductal papillary mucinous neoplasm
- Solid pseudopapillary tumor

Malignant tumors
- Ductal adenocarcinoma
- Intraductal papillary mucinous carcinoma
- Mucinous cystadenocarcinoma
- Signet ring cell carcinoma
- Adenosquamous carcinoma
- Anaplastic carcinoma
- Mixed ductal endocrine carcinoma
- Osteoclast-like giant cell tumor
- Acinar cell carcinoma
- Pancreatoblastoma

- pancreatic neuroendocrine tumors (see page 110)
- pancreatic lymphoma (as an isolated site)
- metastasis to the pancreas (as an isolated site)
- adenocarcinoma of the ampulla of Vater
- intrapancreatic bile duct adenocarcinoma
- duodenal adenocarcinoma.

Pancreatic cancer is one of the most common causes of cancer death in Westernized countries. Worldwide there are approximately 250 000 new cases each year; 70 000 in Europe and 32 000 in the USA. The overall crude incidence of pancreatic cancer is 7.8 per 100 000 population; the peak incidence is in the 65–75-year age group. With an increasingly elderly population, there can be no expectation of a marked reduction in incidence. However, although the overall incidence of pancreas cancer around the world is increasing, in the USA there has been a fall in the total incidence of pancreatic cancer, more so for men than for women.

The majority of patients present with advanced disease and have an overall median survival of less than 6 months, and a 5-year survival rate of 0.4–5%. Between 2.6% and 9% of patients undergo pancreatic resection, with an overall median survival of 11–20 months and a 5-year survival rate of 7–25%; virtually all patients die within 7 years of surgery.

Tobacco smoking is the major risk factor, but the risk is only approximately twofold and accounts for no more than 30% of all cases. The second most important risk factor is a familial background (5–10%). Familial pancreatic cancer is rare, however, although germline mutations of the gene *BRCA2* are found in 10–20% of such families. Other families have a combination of pancreatic cancer and melanoma in which there are germline mutations of the gene p16^{INK4a}. In addition, there are a variety of familial pancreatic cancer syndromes in which the risk of pancreatic cancer is increased significantly:

- Peutz–Jeghers syndrome
- familial breast and ovarian cancer
- familial atypical multiple mole melanoma
- hereditary non-polyposis colon cancer

- ataxia telangiectasia
- Li–Fraumeni syndrome
- familial adenomatous polyposis
- cystic fibrosis.

The risk of pancreatic cancer is increased about fivefold in chronic pancreatitis and fortyfold in hereditary pancreatitis. There is also an association with diabetes mellitus, especially in older patients. Other factors that have weak or unclear roles in the causation of pancreatic cancer include previous surgery, *Helicobacter pylori* infection, pernicious anemia, viral infections, coffee-drinking and a Western diet. Surgery offers the only possibility of cure.

Clinical presentation

In the case of tumors in the head of the pancreas, painless obstructive jaundice (jaundice with dark urine and pale stools) commonly occurs but the presentation is usually insidious.

Symptoms include:
- painless jaundice
- pruritus secondary to jaundice
- fatigue
- weight loss
- back pain (constant, nagging, worse lying down, eased by bending forward and sleeping in sitting position)
- vague dyspepsia or abdominal discomfort
- anorexia
- constipation (reduced food intake)
- steatorrhea (fatty stools)
- late-onset diabetes mellitus without risk factors for diabetes
- acute pancreatitis of unknown cause
- chronic pancreatitis
- acute cholangitis
- vomiting due to duodenal obstruction
- deep-vein thrombosis.

Signs include:
- jaundice
- scratch marks secondary to jaundice
- multiple bruises (ecchymoses) secondary to impaired clotting
- hepatomegaly
- palpable gallbladder – Courvoisier's sign
- cachexia
- left supraclavicular (Virchow's) node enlargement – Troisier's sign
- anemia
- abdominal mass
- metastasis at the umbilicus – Sister Joseph's sign
- ascites
- venous gangrene of the lower limbs
- migratory thrombophlebitis.

Functioning neuroendocrine tumors have their own particular modes of presentation (see Chapter 10, Unusual tumors of the pancreas and ampulla of Vater).

Diagnosis

Radiology. Cancers in the head of the pancreas will cause dilation of both the main bile duct and the main pancreatic duct (97%), giving rise to the classic 'double-duct' radiological sign. Pancreatic cancers are relatively hypovascular, whereas neuroendocrine tumors are hypervascular.

Blood tests should be done for anemia, clotting profile, liver function tests, and proteins.

Serum cancer antigen (CA) 19.9 is a good tumor marker but is artificially elevated in the presence of obstructive jaundice and chronic pancreatitis.

Abdominal ultrasonography is the initial investigation to identify a dilated extrahepatic main bile duct as well as perhaps the primary pancreatic tumor and large liver metastases, if present. This should never be used to exclude a pancreatic cancer.

Contrast-enhanced computed tomography (CT) is the gold standard for diagnosis and staging for resectability. Enlargement of lymph nodes per se is a poor indicator of metastases and hence of resectability. CT is much less accurate in identifying potentially resectable small tumors.

Magnetic resonance imaging (MRI) has similar diagnostic and staging accuracies to that of CT and may have advantages in the detection of liver metastases.

Magnetic resonance cholangiopancreatography may enhance diagnosis by revealing the double-duct sign, and is important for diagnosing and assessing intraductal papillary mucinous neoplasm.

Endoscopic ultrasonography (EUS) is highly sensitive in the detection of small tumors, and small lesions can even be biopsied under EUS guidance. EUS is also useful in staging and is helpful as the next step in evaluating a potentially resectable or equivocally resectable lesion on CT scan.

Endoscopic retrograde cholangiopancreatography (ERCP) is important for the diagnosis of ampullary and duodenal tumors as there is direct visualization, as with EUS, but biopsy is easier, and brush cytology of the bile duct and pancreatic duct may also be undertaken.

Laparoscopy, including laparoscopic ultrasonography, can detect occult metastatic lesions in the liver and peritoneal cavity and is an important adjunct to CT for staging at many centers.

Positron-emission tomography (PET) has not been shown to add anything to the above investigations.

Tissue diagnosis may be obtained by brushings at ERCP or fine-needle aspirations obtained percutaneously or by EUS. CT and EUS-guided fine-needle aspiration have a higher accuracy than ERCP with brush cytology. Preoperative tissue diagnosis may not always be needed in a resectable pancreatic mass if the symptoms, signs, laboratory data and imaging are classical for pancreatic cancer in an otherwise surgically fit patient. However, when a preoperative tissue diagnosis is required in a potentially resectable pancreatic mass, EUS-guided fine-needle aspiration should be the preferred route on account of the lower potential risk of peritoneal seeding, the shorter needle tract and the inclusion of the needle track in the resection specimen (in pancreatic head tumors, the most common pancreatic carcinoma).

Differential diagnosis. In the case of solid lesions, the principal differential diagnoses are focal chronic pancreatitis and periampullary tumors (tumors of the intrapancreatic bile duct, ampulla of Vater and duodenum, and also 'indeterminate' tumors); in the case of cystic tumors they are pancreatic pseudocyst and pheochromocytoma.

Secondary screening

None of these diagnostic tests is appropriate for screening of the general population, but EUS, CT and MRI may be used for secondary screening of high-risk groups, such as in the case of familial pancreatic cancer.

Palliative treatment

All patients with suspected pancreatic cancer must be treated in a specialist high-volume center by a multidisciplinary team. Once the diagnosis is made or strongly suspected, the next objective is to stage the disease. If the tumor is resectable and there are no metastases then resection should be undertaken. If resection is not possible then palliative care should be undertaken (Figure 9.1).

Stenting of the obstructed biliary tree. A stent is inserted through a stricture to relieve the jaundice. If the patient is elderly or has major comorbidities, this is best achieved endoscopically by ERCP. A duodenal stricture may also be stented endoscopically.

Surgical bypass. In younger, fitter patients, biliary bypass is preferred as blockage with stents is avoided. The duodenum is also bypassed – obstruction will occur here in 20% of patients.

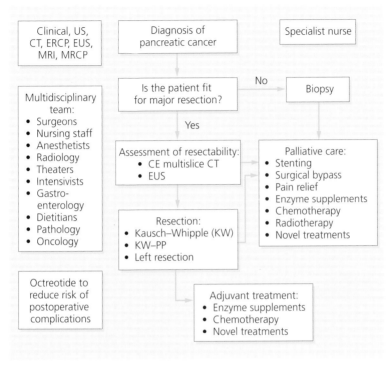

Figure 9.1 Algorithm for the management of patients with pancreatic cancer. CE, contrast-enhanced; CT, computed tomography; ERCP, endoscopic retrograde cholangiopancreatography; EUS, endoscopic ultrasound; FNAB, fine-needle aspiration biopsy; KW-PP, Kausch–Whipple partial pancreatoduodenectomy; LUS, laparoscopic ultrasonography; MRI, magnetic resonance imaging; MRCP, magnetic resonance cholangiopancreatography; US, ultrasonography. Adapted from Ghaneh et al. Pancreatic cancer. In: Williams C, ed. *Evidence-based Oncology*. London: BMJ Books, 2002;247–72.

Pain relief is not easy. A pain team may be needed to advise on the use of opiates, celiac plexus block by percutaneous or EUS-guided route or bilateral transthoracic sympathectomy.

Enzyme supplements are essential, as the main pancreatic duct is usually blocked, leading to pancreatic exocrine insufficiency.

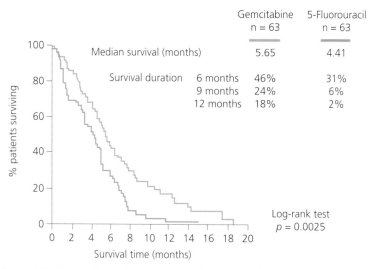

Figure 9.2 The results of the treatment of patients with pancreatic cancer using chemotherapy. $p = 0.0025$ (log-rank test). Adapted from Burris et al. 1997.

Chemotherapy. Monotherapy using gemcitabine has a small survival advantage compared with 5-fluorouracil (or 5-FU) and will also help to reduce pain and weight loss (Figure 9.2). The use of combination therapy with gemcitabine such as erlotinib and capecitabine will improve survival even further.

Radiotherapy in conjunction with chemotherapy may be helpful in controlling pain in patients with locally advanced disease. However, there is no controlled evidence to show that survival is better than with chemotherapy alone.

Curative surgical treatment

Preoperative biliary drainage may be used before surgery to relieve jaundice, in which case metal stents should be avoided as these can make surgery more difficult. The overall mortality for major pancreatic resections is 1–5% in large centers but is much higher otherwise. Postoperative morbidity is high (30–40%), and patients require high-dependency care for at least the first 24 hours after surgery.

Kausch–Whipple partial pancreatoduodenectomy was once the standard procedure for tumors in the head of the pancreas and is still appropriate for large tumors and those close to the pylorus.

Pylorus-preserving partial pancreatoduodenectomy is largely replacing the Kausch–Whipple operation as it does not involve removal of the gastric antrum and pylorus.

Left (distal) partial pancreatectomy includes a splenectomy and is reserved for tumors in the tail of the pancreas.

Total pancreatectomy is reserved for large tumors.

Enucleation is a local resection and is used for small benign neuroendocrine tumors (without metastases) – essentially insulinoma.

Complications

Complications following major pancreatic surgery occur in around 30% of patients and require close monitoring for at least 24 hours (Table 9.2).

TABLE 9.2
Complications of pancreatic surgery

Respiratory complications	10%
Cardiovascular complications	10%
Pancreatic fistula	10%
Delayed gastric emptying	10%
Bleeding	5%
Wound infection	5%
Intra-abdominal abscess	5%
Mortality rate	1–5%
Reoperation rate	5–10%
Reoperative mortality rate	10–30%

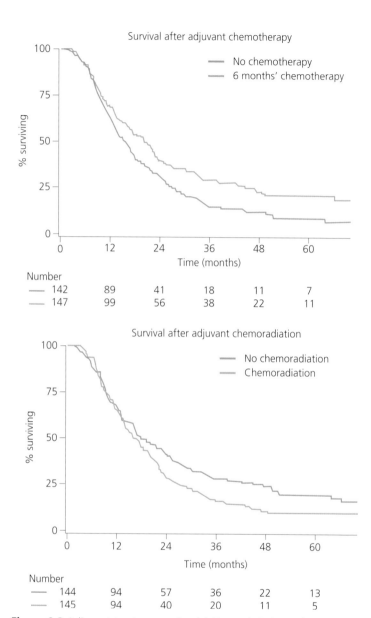

Figure 9.3 Adjuvant treatment using (a) 6 months' chemotherapy (5-fluorouracil and leucovorin) improved survival, whereas (b) chemo-radiation (40 Gy with 5-fluorouracil) did not improve survival in patients with pancreatic cancer. Adapted from Neoptolemos et al. 2004.

TABLE 9.3

Survival rates associated with 6 months' adjuvant treatment following resection

Randomized treatment	Actuarial survival rate	
	2-year	5-year
Observation only	38.7%	10.7%
Chemoradiation	21.7%	7.3%
Chemotherapy	44.0%	29.0%
Chemoradiation followed by chemotherapy	35.5%	13.2%

Chemotherapy consisted of bolus 5-fluorouracil and leucovorin; chemoradiation consisted of 40 Gy plus bolus 5-fluorouracil.
From Neoptolemos et al. 2004. Copyright © 2004 Massachusetts Medical Society. All rights reserved.

Adjuvant treatment

Adjuvant treatment following pancreatic resection is now standard, and should be chemotherapy without the use of radiation. Figure 9.3 illustrates survival rates with 6 months' adjuvant treatment with chemotherapy, which improved survival, or chemoradiotherapy, which did not. Table 9.3 summarizes the survival rates.

Future trends

- Centralization of treatment
- Secondary screening for high-risk groups
- Use of PET in conjunction with CT (fusion PET-CT), an evolving technique that measures the metabolism in tumor cells
- Individual treatment based on molecular characteristics of each tumor and pharmacogenomic constitution of the patient
- Novel biological therapies
- Cancer vaccination
- Anticachexia drugs
- Improved methods of pain control.

Key points – pancreatic cancer

- Pancreatic cancer should be suspected in any older (over 40 years of age) patient with unresolving epigastric symptoms.
- Patients must be managed by a multidisciplinary team in a high-volume regional pancreas cancer center.
- Accurate detection and staging is required with CT and may be supplemented by EUS, CA 19.9 and laparoscopy.
- If the cancer is not resectable, symptoms may be relieved with endoscopic treatment and survival increased with gemcitabine combinations, such as capecitabine.
- Adjuvant chemotherapy should follow resection in order to increase survival.

Key references

Birkmeyer JD, Siewers AE, Finlayson EV et al. Hospital volume and surgical mortality in the United States. *N Engl J Med* 2002;346: 1128–37.

Bruno MJ, Haverkort EB, Tijssen GP et al. Placebo controlled trial of enteric coated pancreatin microsphere treatment in patients with unresectable cancer of the pancreatic head region. *Gut* 1998;42:92–6.

Burris HA 3rd, Moore MJ, Andersen J et al. Improvements in survival and clinical benefit with gemcitabine as first-line therapy for patients with advanced pancreas cancer: a randomized trial. *J Clin Oncol* 1997;15:2403–13.

Coughlin SS, Calle EE, Patel AV, Thun MJ. Predictors of pancreatic cancer mortality among a large cohort of United States adults. *Cancer Causes Control* 2000;11: 915–23.

Hahn SA, Hahn SA, Greenhalf B et al. BRCA2 germ line mutations in familial pancreatic carcinoma. *J Natl Cancer Inst* 2003;95:214–21.

Howes N, Lerch MM, Greenhalf W et al.; European Registry of Hereditary Pancreatitis and Pancreatic Cancer (EUROPAC). Clinical and genetic characteristics of hereditary pancreatitis in Europe. *Clin Gastroenterol Hepatol* 2004;2:252–61.

Jemal A, Murray T, Samuels A et al. Cancer statistics, 2003. *CA Cancer J Clin* 2003;53:5–26.

Malka D, Hammel P, Maire F et al. Risk of pancreatic adenocarcinoma in chronic pancreatitis. *Gut* 2002;51:849–52.

Neoptolemos JP, Stocken DD, Friess H et al. for the members of the European Study Group for Pancreatic Cancer (ESPAC). A randomized trial of chemoradiotherapy and chemotherapy after resection of pancreatic cancer. *N Engl J Med* 2004;350:1200–10.

Sener S, Fremgen A, Menck H, Winchester D. Pancreatic cancer: a report of treatment and survival trends for 100,313 patients diagnosed from 1985–1995, using the National Cancer database. *J Am Coll Surg* 1999;189:1–7.

A variety of tumors arise in close proximity to or within the pancreas that require special consideration and need to be differentiated from pancreatic ductal adenocarcinoma (Table 10.1).

Ampullary, bile duct and duodenal tumors

Epidemiology and pathology. Cancers of the ampulla of Vater, the intrapancreatic bile duct and duodenum are all adenocarcinomas and often present in a manner similar to pancreatic cancer. Bile duct cancers are also called cholangiocarcinomas, although this term is usually reserved for more proximal bile duct tumors. Ampullary tumors arise from the common channel of the ampulla of Vater and are relatively common (around one per 100 000 in the general population) whereas bile duct cancer is much less common and duodenal cancer is rare.

All of these tumors progress from a small benign adenoma through to invasive adenocarcinoma, although most are only detected at the

---

TABLE 10.1

Unusual tumors of or around the pancreas

Tumors arising close to the pancreas
- Adenocarcinoma of the ampulla of Vater
- Intrapancreatic bile duct adenocarcinoma
- Duodenal adenocarcinoma

Unusual tumors of the pancreas
- Cystic tumors of the pancreas
- Intraductal papillary mucinous tumors
- Pancreatic neuroendocrine tumors
- Pancreatic lymphoma (as an isolated site)
- Metastasis to the pancreas (as an isolated site)

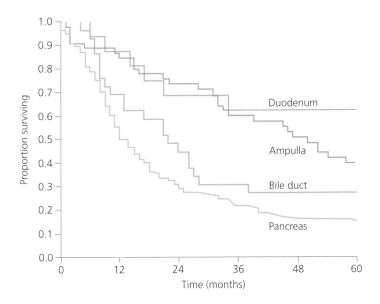

Figure 10.1 Tumor-specific actuarial 5-year survival curves for a cohort of 242 patients treated for periampullary adenocarcinoma by pancreaticoduodenectomy. Adapted from Yeo et al. 1998.

cancerous stage. Ampullary tumors commence as benign adenomas and progress as tubulovillous adenomas before becoming adenocarcinomas. Duodenal tumors also commence as adenomas before progressing to invasive adenocarcinoma. The incidence of duodenal tumors is increased in patients with familial adenomatous polyposis and also Peutz–Jeghers syndrome. The long-term survival of patients with these cancers is much better than that for pancreatic ductal adenocarcinoma (Figure 10.1).

Clinical presentation and diagnosis. These tumors often present in a manner similar to pancreatic cancer, with obstructive jaundice and weight loss. Patients with an ampullary tumor may also present with intermittent jaundice or acute pancreatitis. Patients with duodenal cancer present with iron-deficiency anemia secondary to occult upper gastrointestinal blood loss.

Ampullary and duodenal tumors may be visualized by endoscopic retrograde cholangiopancreatography (ERCP) or endoscopic ultrasonography (EUS), but biopsy is easier with ERCP. Brush cytology of the bile duct may also be undertaken for bile duct strictures using ERCP. Invasive adenocarcinomas usually arise deep within an ampullary tumor. For this reason, endoscopic sphincterotomy through the ampullary tumor needs to be performed and biopsies taken from deep within the tumor.

All three tumor types may mimic pancreatic cancer and vice versa. Pancreatic cancer may invade into or ulcerate the ampulla, giving the appearance of an ampullary cancer; ampullary cancer will invade the duodenum and pancreatic parenchyma, mimicking pancreatic cancer; pancreatic cancer may invade and ulcerate the duodenum, giving the appearance of a duodenal cancer; and invasion of the pancreas is typical of a duodenal cancer. A bile duct cancer may invade the main pancreatic duct, giving rise to the classic double-duct sign of pancreatic cancer; the converse applies to 95% of pancreatic cancers arising in the head or uncinate process of the pancreas.

Treatment and prognosis. Ampullary adenomas can be treated by local ampullectomy using a transduodenal approach or by endoscopic excision. A pancreas-preserving total duodenectomy can be used to treat dysplastic duodenal polyps or benign adenomas, especially in patients with familial adenomatous polyposis.

For cancers of the ampulla, bile duct or duodenum, the treatment of choice is a Kausch–Whipple partial pancreatoduodenectomy. The 5-year survival rates for completely resected tumors are about 50%, 30% and 25% for cancers at the three sites, respectively. Unlike pancreatic cancer, long-term cure is possible in large proportion of patients with these cancers.

Ampullary tumors tend to be slow growing so endoscopic stenting can provide good medium-to-long-term palliation. The role of chemoradiation or chemotherapy for these cancers in either the adjuvant or advanced setting is not established.

Pancreatic cystic tumors

These tumors need to be distinguished from benign pancreatic cysts and in particular from pseudocysts secondary to acute or chronic pancreatitis. Fine-needle aspiration of cysts is of value for cytology: amylase is found in pseudocysts, whereas there is a high level of carcinoembryonic antigen in neoplastic tumors.

Serous cystadenomas are almost invariably benign, usually occur in women and are often left-sided. These tumors are harmless and may be observed serially using computed tomography (CT) or EUS.

Mucinous cystadenomas and cystadenocarcinomas by definition contain mucin. Mucinous cystadenomas are premalignant and, along with cystadenocarcinomas, warrant radical excision.

Intraductal papillary mucinous neoplasms are being recognized increasingly. The pathognomonic features include an irregularly dilated main pancreatic duct containing thick mucus that is readily observed being exuded from the ampulla at ERCP, and one or more irregular cysts.

The cysts develop either from the main pancreatic duct or from side branches. Intraductal papillary neoplasms with main pancreatic duct cysts are more likely to be malignant or progress to malignancy than neoplasms with side-branch cysts. Partial radical resection or even total pancreatectomy is necessary in appropriate patients.

Multiple benign cysts may be a feature of polycystic kidney or renal syndrome, part of the von Hippell–Lindau (VHL) syndrome, or may indicate carrier status of the VHL gene.

Other malignant cystic lesions. A variety of pancreatic malignancies may contain cystic elements, including pancreatic ductal adenocarcinoma and neuroendocrine tumors.

Pancreatic lymphoma

By definition, pancreatic lymphoma is restricted to the pancreas and draining lymph nodes. Resection should be undertaken where possible. Chemotherapy should be tried if this is not feasible, although pancreatic lymphomas respond rather poorly.

Metastases to the pancreas

The pancreas is also a site for the spread of metastases from cancers arising in the abdomen, breast, bronchus or skin. Sometimes these metastases are isolated, in which case radical resection is the treatment of choice. Long-term survival is surprisingly good, particularly for tumors of renal origin.

Pancreatic neuroendocrine tumors

Epidemiology and pathology. Pancreatic neuroendocrine tumors arise from cells in the islet of Langerhans or enterochromaffin-like cells. The prevalence is around 2–4 per 100 000 in the general population. In contrast to most other tumors of the pancreas, these tumors tend to be highly vascular, a feature that is important in making a radiological diagnosis. The tumors may be functioning, secreting specific hormones that produce distinct clinical syndromes, or they may be non-functioning (Table 10.2). They may be sporadic in nature (non-inherited) or be part of an inherited neuroendocrine neoplasia syndrome.

The distinction between benign and malignant neuroendocrine tumors is difficult on histological grounds but is suggested by a high mitotic index. The risk of malignancy increases with tumor size (more than 2–3 cm). The only certain method of establishing malignancy is the detection of lymph-node or hepatic metastases. In principle, insulinomas

TABLE 10.2

Pancreatic neuroendocrine tumors

- Insulinoma
- Gastrinoma
- Non-functioning neuroendocrine tumor
- Carcinoid
- Glucagonoma
- Vasoactive intestinal polypeptide tumor (VIPoma)
- Somatostatinoma
- Pancreatic polypeptide tumor (PPoma)

tend to be benign whereas all other pancreatic neuroendocrine tumors have a high propensity to malignancy.

In general, pancreatic neuroendocrine tumors have a good prognosis, provided complete resection of lymph-node and even hepatic metastases is undertaken. Non-functioning pancreatic neuroendocrine tumors have an unpredictable prognosis, even with surgical resection.

Gastrinomas are also frequently found in the duodenum, and carcinoid tumors occur in the ampulla of Vater.

Functioning pancreatic neuroendocrine syndromes

Insulinoma. The classic presentation is Whipple's triad:
- signs and symptoms of hypoglycemia
- a low blood glucose level at the time the signs and symptoms occur
- disappearance of the signs and symptoms when blood glucose levels are raised.

Typically, faintness, fatigue or even coma occurs with fasting (or vigorous exercise) and is relieved rapidly by eating a snack or drinking a liquid rich in glucose. The diagnosis is based on a very low blood sugar (< 2 mmol/L) and a high level of insulin and C-peptide (indicative of endogenous insulin). The main differential diagnosis is self-administration of insulin.

Gastrinoma causes very high gastric acid secretion, resulting in refractory multiple peptic ulcers, often of a severe nature (Zollinger–Ellison syndrome), and sometimes diarrhea. Commonly there is a history of gastric or duodenal perforation or hemorrhage, necessitating emergency surgery on one or more occasion. The diagnosis is based on finding high gastrin levels (> 100 pg/mL, or > 200 pg/mL after secretin stimulation). Gastrin will also be elevated by histamine H_2-receptor blockers, proton-pump inhibitors or *Helicobacter pylori* infection.

Glucagonoma causes a characteristic necrolytic migratory erythema of the skin, often starting in the groin and perineum, and may also affect the oral mucosa. Other features may include attacks of hyperglycemia, stomatitis, vulvitis, anemia, rash, weight loss, diarrhea and psychiatric disturbances. High plasma glucagon levels are invariably found.

Vasoactive intestinal polypeptide (VIP) tumor. A VIPoma causes watery diarrhea and hypokalemia (Verner–Morrison syndrome). This results in massive intestinal loss of sodium and bicarbonate, leading to hypovolemia, hypokalemia and achlorhydria or metabolic acidosis. There may be impaired glucose tolerance (VIP causes mild insulin resistance) and hypercalcemia. The diagnosis is clinched by high plasma levels of VIP.

Carcinoid tumors only cause symptoms if there is large-volume hepatic metastasis.

Somatostatinoma and pancreatic polypeptide tumor do not cause distinct clinical syndromes and should be distinguished from non-functioning neuroendocrine tumors.

Patients with a suspected pancreatic neuroendocrine tumor require a full hormone screen, which should include chromogrannin A and B levels, which are frequently elevated in non-functioning neuroendocrine tumors. Specific hormone immunohistochemistry of a resected specimen will confirm the type of a functioning neuroendocrine tumor and distinguish this from a non-functioning tumor.

Localization of tumors

Pancreatic neuroendocrine tumors are characterized by high vascularity and somatostatin receptors. Most gastrinomas but only half of insulinomas have somatostatin receptors. These features are important in localizing tumors, which can often be very small. Localization is straightforward in 90% of cases but can be very difficult in the remainder, requiring a range of investigations (Table 10.3).

Inherited pancreatic neuroendocrine tumors

There are four known syndromes and all are inherited in an autosomal-dominant manner. A patient with one of these syndromes requires genetic counseling and appropriate genetic testing. Patients with neuroendocrine tumors need to be managed by a multidisciplinary team that includes specialist endocrinologists, gastroenterologists, radiologists and pancreatic surgeons.

TABLE 10.3

Investigations for localising pancreatic neuroendocrine tumors

- Multidetector computed tomography
- Magnetic resonance imaging
- Somatostatin receptor scintigraphy (octreotide scan)
- Scintigraphy using radiolabelled meta-iodobenzylguanidine
- Endoscopic ultrasonography
- Intraoperative ultrasonography
- Selective pancreatic angiography
- Hepatic portal venous sampling and hormone assay

Multiple endocrine neoplasia type 1 (MEN-1). This is characterized by tumors in the parathyroid and enteropancreatic endocrine tissues and the anterior pituitary (mainly prolactinomas) and is caused by the *MEN1* gene. The typical age at diagnosis is 20–40 years, and penetrance is nearly 100% at 50 years of age. Multiple facial angiofibromas occur in 85% of patients. The spectrum of pancreatic islet tumors is:

- gastrinoma in 25–67%
- insulinomas in 10–34%
- non-functioning tumors, including pancreatic polypeptide tumors (PPomas), in 10–50%
- glucagonomas in 3–8%
- VIPomas in 1–5%
- somatostatinomas in less than 1%.

The major feature is diffuse microadenomatosis, with a tumor diameter ranging from 300 μm to 5 mm, usually associated with one or more larger tumors. Patients with MEN-1 are at increased risk of premature death at a median age of 46–48 years.

von Hippel–Lindau (VHL) disease is a rare disease caused by mutation in the *VHL* gene. Hypervascular neurological (central nervous hemangioblastomas and retinal angiomas), renal (clear-cell carcinomas)

113

and adrenal (pheochromocytomas) tumors are the commonly presenting lesions. Unlike the adrenal tumors associated with VHL, the pancreatic neuroendocrine tumors are usually asymptomatic and non-functioning. Multiple pancreatic cysts are common and are invariably benign. In 12% of cases the pancreas may be the only organ affected. The mean age at detection of pancreatic lesions is 38 years. Endolymphatic sac tumors and multiple pancreatic cysts, both of which are rare in the general population, suggest carrier status. The mean age at death without intervention is 41 years, with the most common cause of death being metastatic renal-cell carcinoma or neurological complications from cerebellar hemangioblastomas.

Neurofibromatosis type 1 (NF-1) is a common inherited autosomal-dominant disorder. It affects about 1 in 3000–4000 live births and is caused by the NF-1 gene. In around 20% of patients the gastrointestinal tract is involved, with hyperplasia of submucosal or myenteric nerve plexuses, gastrointestinal stromal tumors, periampullary carcinoids, pheochromocytomas, periampullary paragangliomas, gastrointestinal adenocarcinomas and, rarely, pancreatic neuroendocrine tumors.

Tuberous sclerosis (TSC) is a rare autosomal-dominant genetic disorder resulting from mutation in the *TSC1* or *TSC2* genes. The major feature is the formation of hamartomas and neoplasms in multiple organs (brain, heart, kidney, skin) and, rarely, pancreatic neuroendocrine tumors.

Treatment

Enucleation. Insulinomas cannot be managed well by medical measures and require removal. Most are benign and the operation performed is simple enucleation.

Radical resection. Pancreatic neuroendocrine tumors other than insulinomas tend to be malignant and require radical excison. Malignancy in insulinoma is indicated by the presence of lymph-node metastases, and a formal pancreatic resection is therefore also required.

Gastrinomas are often multiple and are commonly found in the duodenal wall. Surgical resection is the only procedure that will provide cure with a normal life expectancy.

Proton-pump inhibitors will effectively reduce gastric acid secretion from gastrinomas but will not prevent tumor growth and metastases.

Somatostatin receptor antagonists. The syndromes associated with all of these tumors, except for insulinoma, can be managed medically during the wait for surgery (or if there is metastatic disease) with a long-acting somatostatin receptor antagonist.

Surgical tumor debulking is commonly undertaken, since the symptoms may still be difficult to control with somatostatin receptor antagonists.

Radionuclide therapy. Metastatic tumors that can be imaged by somatostatin receptor scintigraphy can be treated by radionuclide tagged to the somatostatin analog. An alternative is the use of radiolabeled meta-iodobenzylguanide (MIBG), a catecholamine analog. Pancreatic neuroendocrine tumors express active amine precursor uptake-1 mechanisms that can internalize MIBG, resulting in its incorporation into cytoplasmic neurosecretory granules.

Chemotherapy. Pancreatic neuroendocrine tumors respond disappointingly to chemotherapy. However, chemotherapy may be useful for patients with poorly differentiated neuroendocrine tumors with a high proliferation index.

Screening
Screening is indicated in patients with inherited pancreatic neuroendocrine tumors to identify pancreatic and extrapancreatic tumors in order to permit timely medical and surgical intervention.

Future trends
- Improved preoperative classification to permit more accurate decision-making regarding operative intervention

- Molecular profiling to enable accurate distinction between tumor types
- Specific medical treatments for the different tumor types
- Improved surveillance in patients with inherited pancreatic neuroendocrine tumors.

Key points – unusual tumors of the pancreas and ampulla of Vater

- Tumor types that occur in the head of the pancreas may have a much better prognosis than the common type of pancreatic cancer.
- Solitary metastases to the pancreas may be worth resecting.
- Patients with neuroendocrine tumors need to be managed by a multidisciplinary team.
- Hypervascular tumors are likely to be neuroendocrine tumors.
- Neuroendocrine tumors should usually be removed surgically.
- Patients with inherited neuroendocrine tumors require genetic counseling and long-term follow-up for pancreatic and other tumor types.

Key references

Alexakis N, Connor S, Ghaneh P et al. Hereditary pancreatic endocrine tumours. *Pancreatology* 2004;4: 417–35.

Brandi M, Gagel R, Angeli A et al. Guidelines for diagnosis and therapy of MEN type 1 and type 2. *J Clin Endocrinol Metab* 2001;86:5658–71.

Brugge WR, Lauwers GY, Sahani D et al. Cystic neoplasms of the pancreas. *N Engl J Med* 2004; 351:1218–26.

Chari ST, Yadav D, Smyrk TC et al. Study of recurrence after surgical resection of intraductal papillary mucinous neoplasm of the pancreas. *Gastroenterology* 2002;123:1500–7.

Norton J, Fraker D, Alexander H et al. Surgery to cure the Zollinger–Ellison syndrome. *N Engl J Med* 1999;341:635–44.

Thompson N. Current concepts in the surgical management of multiple endocrine neoplasia type 1 pancreatic duodenal disease. Results in the treatment of 40 patients with Zollinger–Ellison syndrome, hypoglycaemia or both. *J Intern Med* 1998;243:495–500.

Yeo CJ, Sohn TA, Cameron JL et al. Periampullary adenocarcinoma: analysis of 5-year survivors. *Ann Surg* 1998;227:821–31.

Useful resources

American Gastroenterological
Association
7910 Woodmont Avenue, 7th floor
Bethesda, MD 20814, USA
Tel: +1 301 654 2055
Fax: +1 301 652 3890
www.gastro.org

American Pancreas Association
www.american-pancreatic-
association.org

American Society for Clinical
Oncology (ASCO)
www.asco.org/ac/

British Society of
Gastroenterology
3 St Andrew's Place, Regent's Park
London NW1 4LB, UK
Tel: +44 (0)20 7387 3534
Fax: +44 (0)20 7487 3734
www.bsg.org.uk

CancerBACUP (UK)
3 Bath Place
Rivington Street
London EC2A 3JR, UK
Freephone UK helpline:
 0808 800 1234
Helpline: +44 (0)20 7739 2280
Tel (office): +44 (0)20 7696 9003
Fax: +44 (0)20 7696 9002
www.cancerbacup.org.uk/cancertyp
e/pancreas

Cancer Help UK
Cancer Information Department
Cancer Research UK
PO Box 123, Lincoln's Inn Fields
London WC2A 3PX, UK
cancer.info@cancer.org.uk
www.cancerhelp.org.uk/help/defaul
t.asp?page=2795

EUROPAC

The European Register for Familial Pancreas Cancer and Hereditary Pancreatitis (the principal register in Europe providing advice and research in inherited pancreatic disorders)
EUROPAC Co-ordinator
School of Cancer Studies
Royal Liverpool University Hospital
Liverpool L69 3GA, UK
europac@liv.ac.uk
www.liv.ac.uk/surgery/europac.html

National Cancer Institute (USA)

www.cancer.gov/cancertopics/types/pancreatic

National Pancreas Foundation (USA)

364 Boylston Street, 4th Floor
Boston, MA02116, USA
www.pancreasfoundation.org

Pancreas Cancer Web (USA)

Johns Hopkins University
www.path.jhu.edu/pancreas

Pancreas.org (USA)

www.pancreas.org

Pancreas Web

www.pancreasweb.com

Pancreatica (USA)

Lorenzen Cancer Foundation
149 Bonifacio Place
Monterey, CA 93940, USA
www.pancreatica.org

Pancreatic Cancer Action Network (PanCAN) (USA)

www.pancan.org/Healthcare/index.html

Pancreatic Cancer UK

31 Brooklyn Drive, Emmer Green
Reading RG4 8SR, UK
enquiries@pancreaticcancer.org.uk
www.pancreaticcancer.org.uk

Index

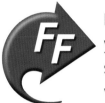

Imagine if every time you wanted to know something you knew where to look...

Over one million copies sold

- Written by world experts
- Concise and practical
- Up to date
- Designed for ease of reading and reference
- Copiously illustrated with useful photographs, diagrams and charts.

Our aim is to make *Fast Facts* the world's most respected medical handbook series. Feedback on how to make titles even more useful is always welcome (feedback@fastfacts.com).

More than 70 *Fast Facts* titles, including:

Asthma	Inflammatory Bowel Disease (second edition)
Benign Prostatic Hyperplasia (fifth edition)	Irritable Bowel Syndrome (second edition)
Bipolar Disorder	Liver Disorders
Bladder Cancer (second edition)	Menopause (second edition)
Bleeding Disorders	Minor Surgery
Brain Tumors	Multiple Sclerosis (second edition)
Breast Cancer (third edition)	Osteoporosis (fourth edition)
Chronic Obstructive Pulmonary Disease	Parkinson's Disease
Colorectal Cancer (second edition)	Prostate Cancer (fourth edition)
Contraception (second edition)	Psoriasis (second edition)
Dementia	Renal Disorders
Depression (second edition)	Respiratory Tract Infection (second edition)
Dyspepsia (second edition)	Rheumatoid Arthritis
Eczema and Contact Dermatitis	Schizophrenia (second edition)
Endometriosis (second edition)	Sexual Dysfunction
Epilepsy (third edition)	Sexually Transmitted Infections
Erectile Dysfunction (third edition)	Skin Cancer
Gynecological Oncology	Smoking Cessation
Headaches (second edition)	Soft Tissue Rheumatology
Hyperlipidemia (third edition)	Thyroid Disorders
Hypertension (third edition)	Urinary Stones

Orders

To order via the website, or to find regional distributors, please go to www.fastfacts.com

For telephone orders, please call +44 (0)1752 202301 (Europe), 1 800 247 6553 (USA, toll free) or +1 419 281 1802 (Americas)